6616 155.937 WRI

✗

D1392194

Sudden Death
Intervention Skills
for the Caring
Professions

Sudden Death
Intervention Skills for
the Caring Professions

Bob Wright SRN RMN
Clinical Nurse Specialist (Crisis Care)
Accident and Emergency Department
Leeds General Infirmary
Leeds

Churchill Livingstone
EDINBURGH LONDON MELBOURNE AND NEW YORK 1991

CHURCHILL LIVINGSTONE
Medical Division of Longman Group UK Limited

Distributed in the United States of America by Churchill Livingstone Inc., 1560 Broadway, New York, N.Y. 10036, and by associated companies, branches and representatives throughout the world.

First published 1991

ISBN 0-443-04133-4

British Library Cataloguing in Publication Data
Wright, Bob
  Sudden death: intervention skills for the caring professions.
  1. Medicine. Nursing
  I. Title
  610.7361

Library of Congress Cataloging in Publication Data
Wright, Bob, SRN, RMN.
    Sudden death: intervention skills for the caring professions/Bob Wright.
      p.   cm.
    Includes bibliographical references.
    ISBN 0–443–04133–4
    1. Sudden death. I. Title.
    [DNLM: 1. Crisis Intervention — methods. 2. Death, Sudden.
WM 401 W947s]
RC86.7.W75   1991
155.9'37 — dc20
DNLM/DLC
for Library of Congress

Produced by Longman Singapore Publishers (Pte) Ltd.
Printed in Singapore

Acknowledgements

I am indebted to my friend, Marjorie Ashdown, who did so much work with the relatives of sudden death victims. Her contribution was not only an integral part of the study, but a major one.

I am also aware that hers was, at times, a stressful role, and we were both eager to share our involvement in all the aspects of the deaths from the beginning to where we left them.

I developed my role as a workshop facilitator, teacher and speaker alongside Marjorie, whose wide experience in this field gave me both knowledge and encouragement.

My friends and colleagues at work have had to put up with my preoccupation with the study, and have willingly participated. I am so grateful that they fed and encouraged my enthusiasm.

My wife, Fiona, is a great support to me both personally and professionally. This involves not only having to listen to me, but also to the occasional frantic phone call in the middle of the night. Whilst I was locked away writing, my children were heard to say:

'Oh no, not death again.'

Anne not only typed this but drew diagrams, re-arranged it and at times made sense of it. Her help and enthusiasm for the book were a great asset.

Last, but by no means least, I must thank all those people whose response to and encounter with sudden death taught me so much. Those seen for the study all gave written permission for the material and statistics to be used.

Leeds 1991   B. W.

Contents

Contents

Introduction

This book concludes a study of sudden death begun 5 years ago by Marjorie Ashdown and myself. It was started in response to the nursing staff in the Accident and Emergency Department at Leeds General Infirmary who needed to have the care of the families of sudden death victims evaluated.

We looked at 100 sudden deaths and carefully recorded the details of the circumstances of the death, the care of the family, and the family's response in the hours surrounding the immediate loss. The nurse caring for the family and friends was asked to evaluate the family's response to the loss at the immediate time of the loss, and also to describe the aspects the nurse herself had difficulty with.

We wrote to the families 6 months and 10 months later, and asked to visit them. We asked them to describe what happened to them at the hospital, and to discuss positive and negative aspects of the immediate care. We then attempted to link this care with how they had adjusted and adapted in the long term.

The long-term implications of the immediate care were discussed. Many of the families were able to describe in some detail both the care received and their response to that very painful day in their lives. The responses were enlightening, moving, and have much to teach us about the human condition and some of the difficulties of our work. The insights received have been invaluable.

I want to begin with a problem. It is important to me that you allow me to begin here because it illustrates the difficulty in beginning this book and the way the contents are set out.

Part of my study of sudden death was to focus on and ident- ify the emotional responses from the relatives which produce the greatest difficulties for us the carers. The theory is that if we are able to work more effectively with these difficulties then we, the carers, will emerge feeling less drained and damaged by our caring.

I could have begun with listing these difficulties, and how we might respond. This would seem logical in that we discard or attack the difficulties first, thus leaving the way clear to begin describing positive and useful caring skills. This is often an expectation of the workshops I run dealing with the problems of coping with sudden death. Those of you who know of our initial reluctance to even attempt to care will know what I mean:

'What on earth can I do?'

The struggle, and often the accompanying pain and anguish, in that initially overwhelming grief is, perhaps, one reason to welcome this order of topics. But on closer consideration I found that this approach would not suit the overall plan be- cause I feel I must begin with my frailty and difficulties. My struggle, my fumbling for the right words, my dissatisfaction with my performance and effectiveness is the beginning. There are lessons to be learnt from our struggle to care, to get it right, and to contribute something in a most difficult and overwhelming life crisis.

I have begun therefore with interventions which we know about and which I have found useful.

These structured approaches offer some order and parameters in a scenario that is potentially quite the opposite, i.e. chaotic, disordered, overwhelming and with far-reaching implications. Armed with this theory, we can enter reality.

The awesome impact of the event is the facing of reality. Anything we learn about this will be learnt from our struggles and difficulties. I believe you will be reading this because you have been in that position and want to be useful, comforting, and to have on offer something those people stricken with grief will value. The way in which our contribution to the event is perceived by the grieving can teach us a lot.

We are witness to an event that cannot be equalled in its ability to impose emotional pain and distress on another person. The loss of a significant loved one is said to be the most difficult life event that can be experienced. Yet many individuals manage to live with and emerge from the experience continuing to live their lives. So, if we can contribute to this successful re-emergence (and I believe we can) we will have made a very special contribution.

This is not about something magical or mystical, it is about using the event and all its pain and difficulties on impact, time and time again. The things we can do or offer cannot be imposed on people, but can facilitate the start of that process we call grief, which is necessary if one is to re-emerge from bereavement. Grieving is a process that begins on the news of a sudden death and whilst the uniqueness of each event is striking there are still opportunities to gain experience and understanding that will help equip us to care for others in the same position.

So the stresses of caring, and the way we might tackle them, are at the end of the book. Our difficulties and search to offer something positive are near the start.

I return, then, to the beginning; and we begin with the awful impact of the event and our hesitations and wonderings before we face it. We begin with our fear and trepidation at confronting the bereaved, with our struggling to find a voice and words as we enter a room and say:

'Mrs Jones. I am sorry. I have some bad news . . .'

It may be that later you are in the position to say:

'How can I help you with this?'

while secretly, thinking, 'Yes, *how* can I help you with this?' With sudden death it will be apparent that the pain is sharp and devastating. It will produce bewilderment, protest, fight and flight. Its implications will take the grief-stricken over their lives with the deceased, how far they had come with them and where they were going with them. This will demand some sense being made out of something senseless and outrageous. It will immobilise or energise and produce erratic and disordered behaviour. Some will literally want to crawl up the wall or into a corner.

When you are confronted with all this, you will feel the need to try to do something useful. This need has brought you here now. You will want, as I do, to feel effective, useful and comforting. The need to feel effective is not just for your clients but for you. In working with such extremes of distress, our sense of having something positive to offer will help us to leave it behind. The ability to disengage from it is important.

Our resourcefulness in dealing with these difficulties stems from our vulnerability and our humanity and it is that which helps us to interact and make the interaction meaningful. So we begin as in reality, with the chaos and the crisis, and its awesome confrontation. We will look at the struggle to replace pain and fragmentation with wholeness and the attempts to restore order.

My involvement in all this requires some explanation. The impact of loss has been a major focus of my working life. Twenty five years ago I worked for 3 years at St George's Crypt in the city of Leeds. Here, beneath the city centre church, slept up to 100 homeless men. Night after night they lay on benches within the vaults, some on tombs the contents of which had been exhumed and re-interred to make way for the living.

The men in this sad group were isolated and often damaged by loss. Some of the losses had produced mistrust and fear of re-bonding. Trust and intimacy can be too risky — you might get hurt. Some of the resultant anger and guilt produced by the losses separated these men from family and friends, and the welfare system. Wars, divorce, separation, illness and injury had taken their toll. The years of isolation and pre-occupation with pain and injustice had resulted in some badly damaged people.

It occurred to me on many occasions that much pain could have been prevented with the right amount of care and support at the time of the loss. I understand that this is only part of the answer — flight and its ensuing isolation are difficult to work with and so are some angry and mistrustful individuals. Some people are difficult to love and care for.

The resulting suspicion, resentment and overt paranoia

make this group of men difficult to form relationships with. It can nevertheless be done, and they taught me a great deal about the value of immediate care and about the resulting long-term difficulties if this care is ineffective.

From here, I did 3 years' psychiatric nurse training and then worked in the acute area of psychiatry. When I went on to do general nurse training I took with me an awareness of our vulnerability due, in part, to this background. I returned to acute psychiatry and spent 2 years training in basic counselling, marital counselling and group work skills. Fourteen years ago I obtained a post as charge nurse in the Accident and Emergency Department at Leeds General Infirmary.

Leeds General Infirmary is a major accident centre and a regional neurosurgical unit. Many critically ill patients, with serious head injuries, arrive in our resuscitation room from other hospitals, for neurosurgical evaluation and intervention. Many relatives have made that journey with the patient, or followed in a police car, or have driven themselves to the hospital desperate for some miracle. Other patients arrive critically ill having collapsed at home or in the street. For many families it is just another day that becomes one of enormous significance, a day which is to change their lives. Whilst I have no illusions about putting everything right for them, I feel there is a great significance in our management of the immediate care, both for the bereaved and for us.

Awareness of the true meaning of the event, and some sensitive and sustained care is of real value, not only at that time but in the long term. I feel we can help the bereaved begin that process we call grief and make use of the events in the immediate term to begin some process that will heal. The immediate care takes time and commitment.

Initially my work was to look at crisis intervention in the Accident and Emergency Department. To widen my research area I went to the USA to work with crisis intervention nurses in Boston and New York, and later to Israel. My completed study was later published under the title *Caring in Crisis*, the third chapter of which dealt in more detail with the crisis of sudden death. It was from this base that a more detailed study began. The nurses I was working with also had a strong sense of the value of the immediate care of the suddenly bereaved. They were not content simply to experience this feeling; happily they were able to make strong statements about its difficulties:

'I was not prepared properly to do this work.'

'You tell me it is useful but how do I know?'

'Sometimes I feel that every time I am in that situation I lose a part of me. Tell me it's worth it.'

'I can face the most horrific multiple injuries and the stresses of the resuscitation room, but please don't ask me to go to the relatives when the patient dies — that's even worse.'

It appeared that the questions being asked were about us gaining some insights into our contribution to the situation, and its value. The underlying message seemed to be:

'Tell me the value of this work and equip me to handle it. That insight will give me the strength and some ability to get in there and do it well.'

One thing we all want to be is effective. This helps us to step where angels fear to. It was some of these questions, and the need to gain knowledge and insight into the needs of the suddenly bereaved, that prompted me to begin this study.

1

The crisis of sudden death

Barbara was trying to sort this thing out in her head and it didn't make any sense. Her boss had told her that Richard had been injured in an accident and that she had to ring the hospital. She must ring at once, he had said, it was serious. Suddenly everyone in the office was looking at her. She didn't want all this attention. What did they want her to do? None of this made sense. He had been all right when he dropped her off at the office; he was always in a hurry.

'This is a real nuisance, he knows how busy we are on Mondays. I hope he's not hurt. It can't be that serious.' She heard herself telling her friend, 'Please tell me it isn't.'

She was shaking when she heard the voice answer 'Accident and Emergency' and then the voice said it was serious and she was to come at once. 'Bring a friend or a relative with you,' the voice had suggested.

Her friend, Jackie, offered to drive her there, and as she drove towards the hospital, Jackie told Barbara not to worry. 'Worry! Why should I?' Barbara thought. 'We have been married one year. Richard's had a serious accident, and she says don't worry. Good job he's tough and has determination. Plays rugby for the local pub. Older, weaker people have a terrible time getting over accidents.'

As they pulled up at the hospital, Jackie was still talking to her, and Barbara realised she hadn't heard a word her friend had said.

The nurse showed her into a little room and asked her to sit down.

'How is he?' Barbara asked.

'I am Julie Watson, one of the staff nurses here.'

'For God's sake, answer me,' Barbara thought.

'I am sorry, but your husband Richard has been very seriously injured in a car accident. He has serious multiple injuries and we are very concerned about the seriousness of his injuries. A team of doctors are trying to save him. His life is in danger.'

'In danger,' Barbara thought. 'Is he dying?' she asked with a voice that was barely audible.

'No, don't be silly,' Jackie, her friend, said. 'Of course he isn't.'

The nurse stopped her. 'It is very serious and that is a possibility. Do you want any of your family here, or anyone else?'

'No,' Barbara said firmly, 'Not yet. I don't want to upset my parents.'

'What about his?' asked the nurse.

'Let's wait,' Barbara replied. 'He only has his mother and she has a weak heart. We don't want to upset her.'

The nurse left the room saying she was going to get more information.

As soon as the nurse had left, Jackie said, 'She could have put it a nicer way instead of being so blunt. Drink this awful tea they've given you. When we visited my grandmother here it was like that then. We sat with her for two days whilst she was dy . . . Sorry Barbara. She seemed awfully young that nurse, to be telling you those things.'

'Shut up,' Barbara thought, trying to block out Jackie's voice. 'This doesn't make any sense. There we were this morning, saying it was only a month since we got back from Spain, and how it seemed months ago, and talking about where we would go next. This isn't right. I've not done anything wrong.'

The nurse came back into the room. Jackie's voice was silenced and Barbara realised she hadn't heard a single word Jackie had seen saying.

'I am sorry Barbara, but he is worse,' the nurse told her. 'The main thing we are worried about is his serious head injury. The neurosurgeons are here and they are taking him to the theatre for a scan.'

'I don't want him to be a cabbage,' Barbara protested, and then quickly apologised for having said it. Then she burst into tears and said, 'I just want him to live.'

The nurse held her hand and said nothing. Barbara was glad of this. She just wanted some peace and quiet. She felt so helpless, and wondered if she should be doing or saying something, and desperately searched around inside her head for an answer to it all. There must be some way of putting it right. Perhaps she hadn't really woken up this morning. Perhaps it was all a dream. Yes, of course. She smiled quietly to herself, and remembered the relief when you realise how stupid you are to believe the nightmare could be true.

Jackie and the nurse were looking at her in a puzzled way, and were beginning to look helpless themselves.

'What are you thinking?' the nurse asked Barbara.

'I'm just thinking this cannot be true. It's all a bad dream. Soon I will wake up. Is he any better? I don't want him to die. He's all I have. I love him so much. Go and see. I'm all right here. Go and help, you might be needed. Don't worry about me.'

Jackie was twisting her handkerchief round and round into a big knot. She asked Barbara for the second time whether it would not be better if her mother or father were here.

'No it would not,' Barbara answered firmly. 'It's not that bad yet, is it? Is it? Tell me it isn't.'

Barbara felt weak, helpless and frustrated. 'Go back to the office, I'm all right.' She paused, her voice faltering. 'I'm sorry, don't leave me.'

Barbara clung to her friend and cried.

Jackie told her she'd be all right. When the nurse came back she looked serious and seemed to lose her voice for a moment. She cleared her throat.

'He's no better, Barbara. I'm sorry. Things are looking very bad. Are you sure about not getting your parents? You need someone close to you at a time like this.'

'Yes, all right then,' Barbara replied. 'But how do I tell them. This is so awful for them. It's not right.'

The nurse offered to tell them, and left the room to telephone. Barbara hoped she would do it gently and that her father would drive carefully to the hospital and not start shouting at her mother. Jackie prayed that they would come soon. Why did she always find herself in these situations? Then immediately she felt guilty for thinking such a thing.

Barbara was remembering the first time she met Richard, when she thought he was talking too loudly, but decided he was doing it just to get some attention. That was 3 years ago. It seemed just like yesterday in some ways, yet in other ways a lifetime.

'We've been here well over an hour now,' she heard Jackie saying, 'You'd think they'd tell us something.'

The door opened and Julie, the staff nurse, came in, followed by a doctor. Barbara looked for signs of hope on their faces but did not see any.

'Mrs Morris?' the doctor asked. 'Mrs Barbara Morris? Is your husband Richard Morris?'

'Yes, yes, what do you want to say?'

'I am sorry to have to tell you that your husband has just died.'

Barbara looked round at each of them, about to protest, but no words came out.

'He had very serious injuries and, despite all our efforts we were unable to save him,' the doctor continued. 'I am very sorry. Is there anything you want to ask me?'

The doctor waited. After a few minutes Barbara asked 'Was he in pain? What did he know?'

The doctor quickly assured her that Richard would have known nothing about the accident, and Jackie was nodding her head in agreement.

Barbara did not hear the doctor saying he was leaving now, but would come back and talk to her later if she wanted. She just saw him going out of the door. Her head was a mass of questions: none of it made any sense. How can it be that this morning I was married to a man called Richard, everything was fine, and now he is dead and I am a widow. I do not even have his child. We have only just started our lives. We have things to do. It is not right. Why? Why?

Just then, her mother walked through the door, followed by her father.

'He's dead, Mum,' Barbara said, 'Dad, he's dead.'

There can be no other life event that has the same impact as sudden death. Holmes & Rahe (1967) were able to identify which life crisis produced the most difficulty, not only on impact but in the long term. I was not surprised at what was at the top of the list but as a carer working with issues around loss it is of special interest to note the other crises which come closest to it. If any of these other crises occur at the same time of the sudden death it will compound the loss and more powerfully incapacitate the person. To imagine this event becoming part of our lives is a mammoth task. For most people it is too difficult to contemplate. How do we begin to understand the impact this loss can have on the many aspects of our lives?

As nurses one of our difficulties in working with sudden death must be the awareness of its strength, enormity and complexity. Many people will have pondered on what they would do if it happened to them, but then quickly decide that this is an exercise to be avoided.

Perhaps we cannot live life to the full if we acknowledge the thought that a loved one can be taken from us suddenly. Perhaps there is little use in giving it any thought? If it happens, well, then we have to deal with it.

So our ambivalent feelings towards sudden death present another difficulty in working with it — the problems become ours as well as our client's. 'What can we do about it?' is the question posed by a sudden death, but an underlying instinct is also to keep away from it.

The shock and disbelief have much more impact than has an anticipated death. In his study of young widows/widowers in the Harvard Bereavement Study, Parkes (1975) was able to identify that in sudden death, there was clearly a more emotionally disturbed response. The disturbance persisted throughout the first year of bereavement.

Another study (Lundin 1984), which followed up significant relatives 8 years after a death, found that where death was unexpected, feelings of remorse, self-reproach and distress were more marked than in those who had experienced an anticipated death.

Some sudden deaths produce even more problems than others. Sudden infant death syndrome (SIDS) or cot deaths

Table 1.1 Social readjustment rating scale (reprinted with permission from Holmes & Rahe. Journal of Psychosomatic Research 1967 11: 213–218 © Pergamon Press plc).

Life event	Mean value
1. Death of spouse	100
2. Divorce	73
3. Marital separation from mate	65
4. Detention in jail or other institution	63
5. Death of a close family member	63
6. Major personal injury or illness	53
7. Marriage	50
8. Being fired at work	47
9. Marital reconciliation with mate	45
10. Retirement from work	45
11. Major change in the health or behavior of a family member	44
12. Pregnancy	40
13. Sexual difficulties	39
14. Gaining a new family member (e.g. through birth, adoption, older person moving in)	39
15. Major business readjustment (e.g. merger, reorganization, bankruptcy)	39
16. Major change in financial state (e.g. a lot worse off or a lot better off than usual)	38
17. Death of a close friend	37
18. Changing to a different line of work	36
19. Major change in the number of arguments with spouse (e.g. either a lot more or a lot less than usual regarding childbearing, personal habits)	35
20. Taking out a mortgage or loan for a major purchase (e.g. for a home, business)	31
21. Foreclosure on a mortgage or loan	30
22. Major change in responsibilities at work (e.g. promotion, demotion, lateral transfer)	29
23. Son or daughter leaving home (e.g. marriage, attending college)	29
24. Trouble with in-laws	29
25. Outstanding personal achievement	28

lead to some very serious difficulties in the grieving process. I have seen several parents who have described themselves as being 'stuck' with some pain or difficulty. This standstill, or inability to leave some painful focus, can be with them for years.

Raphael (1984) describes the relentless search for the cause of death. Parents blame each other, and the role of the police and ensuing enquiries produce defensiveness and mis-understanding. Peppers & Knapp (1980) suggest that for most mothers the grief remains with them for the rest of their lives. They do not say it is persistently present but call it 'shadow grief,' describing it as a recurrent intrusion that casts a shadow across life. It is a transient reminder that, on occasions, produces a painful memory of loss and can shut out the joy of an occasion. They describe this transient reminder of the loss as a burden the mother must bear for the rest of her life.

Whilst you would expect the death of a child to be more problematical, where the death was anticipated the parents do not show more psychiatric symptoms than would be expected in any other kind of death. A study by Shanfield et al (1986) showed that in the anticipated death of a child, half of the parents reported a sense of personal growth and a great de-gree of intimacy with the rest of the family. Far worse outcomes were reported where the cause of death of the child was a road traffic accident. The difficulties were more marked for the mother than the father.

Anticipatory grief work may well have a better outcome, if the one who knows what the end result will be does not deny or suppress this knowledge. This may be done to avoid up-setting the dying person or other family members, but the point of death can then have all the hallmarks of a sudden death.

Death by suicide has, in my experience of counselling, resulted in some extremely difficult issues and must cause some very poor outcomes, as will deaths by violence. Sudden death in these cases is not only a violation of the ones left behind but also a violation of their belief in life itself.

Wordon (1983) describes how anticipatory grief refers to the grieving that occurs prior to the actual loss. Many deaths occur with some warning, and during this period of anticipation, the survivor begins some of the tasks of mourning, and begins to experience some of the grief. Wordon goes on to describe how, in sudden death, the prolonged grieving can produce resentment which leads to guilt.

The term anticipatory grief was first used in the classic paper by Lindemann (1944) which by now must have been read by all who have studied the crisis of sudden death. Lindemann refers to the absence of overt signs of grief at the time of the loss, by survivors of the Coconut Grove Club fire. This numbness and personal difficulty with their own response is often apparent on impact of death:

'How do you expect me to respond?'
'I do not know how I should feel.'

Sudden death, then, we know from the experience of others, has the capacity to leave people damaged or to result in a prolonged and painful grieving process. The lack of time or preparation for the death leaves so much unfinished. This in turn leads to a double kind of grief — grief for what is lost and grief for what might have been.

There will usually be areas in the relationship that have been unrealised, areas that had greater potential. There will be unresolved emotional issues where, if there had been warning about potential loss, validation of feelings and confirmation of strengths in the relationship could have been given. The grief for themselves, and what might have been, is therefore inevitably an issue to discuss.

Grief for the deceased, what he has missed, his lack of time, and the injustice of this, compounds 'what might have been' for the bereaved:

'He was young and vital, so full of life. He never knew what it was like to fall in love or be a father.'

The many faces of sudden death give it a breadth and length that demand great concentration and energy. What is lost and what might have been are just two of the issues that must be discussed. All the issues involved are very time-consuming to deal with, and use up lots of energy. Some bereaved people describe themselves as being fed up with the whole thing, and lack the commitment to focus on or continue to work on the problem. They want answers, and some spend long periods in involved exploration of the issues. This often comes to an abrupt halt, holding up the process of grieving or prolonging it. The grief process becomes drawn out, imponderable and overwhelming.

When this happens it takes some effort, patience, skill and determination to work with it. By skill, I mean that some discipline and ability are needed to discover what stage this person has reached in his grief, and to make it manageable for him. We need to examine ways of breaking grief down into manageable components in the immediate and the long term. The ways suggested in this first chapter are not blueprints for achieving clear and unequivocal outcomes, they are simply an offering of what may be useful in your work with sudden death. They may offer pathways to making sudden death manageable by decreasing its impact and potential to damage.

The whole issue of preventative medicine and its value in our health care system is another topic. Glick et al (1974) demonstrate clearly how people with grief responses may present it in the (to them) more acceptable form as illness. Many of the young widows in this study had increased visits to doctors within the first year of loss, with upper respiratory tract infections or gynaecological problems. This group, compared with a control group, had a higher incidence of these problems.

In our Accident and Emergency Department, I have witnessed the difficulty of where the real focus of health care problems lies: many people with unresolved loss present with vague chest pains and panic attacks.

Preventative medicine is low down on the list of health care priorities. Effective and committed intervention at the time of sudden death and afterwards must greatly reduce the incidence of illness and injury resulting from this crisis. Raphael (1980) demonstrates how specific programmes on high risk groups can effectively intervene. She discusses (1984) how intervention is important both on impact and over time, in helping people come to terms with their loss.

An investigation into why sudden death produces particular difficulties in grieving will also focus on the difficulties of working with the problem. For example, the overall protracted period of mourning and grieving is reflected in our counselling of the bereaved person. Some of this counselling will be drawn out, may come to a halt, and may contain many of the same components as experienced on the impact of grief.

Therefore, our expectations, when discussed with the client, must be realistic. We will return to some of the determinants of grief as described by Parkes (1975) towards the end of this chapter. These are a useful check list to help the client identify an area of difficulty or avoidance.

Before we do that, I would like to examine other structured ways of intervening in the crisis of sudden death:

The first one involves holistic principles and is not only a philosophy underlying all my interventions, but a useful way of examining human dynamics. The five dimensions used in holistic counselling cover the many facets of the person closely involved in a sudden death and, I feel, usefully break down and identify problems.

HOLISTIC PRINCIPLES

The principles are established to provide a framework that will enhance the carer/client relationship in many settings. The focus is on five human dimensions (Box 1.1) and was developed by Herbert Otto in the early 1970s.

```
1. Physical
2. Emotional
3. Intellectual
4. Social
5. Spiritual
```

Box 1.1 Five dimensions in holism.

This approach to treatment or therapy may be used by all therapists regardless of their theoretical orientation. Despite the many approaches and areas of focus, holism makes assumptions that are common to all people. Although many methods and theories abound, holism recognises that everyone has unrealised potential. This is best developed through self-responsibility and self-help.

People who have been affected by a sudden death will talk about a loss of control over their lives and about powerlessness or helplessness. One of our goals should be to help people regain control and power whilst giving them the freedom and space to express the pain of death.

Holism looks at the difficulties of being human and the concern for the individual's existence, rather than at theories on human nature. There is a premise that inner experience provides people with insights or their own sense of meaning and purpose, and that individuals make choices throughout life for which they are personally responsible.

I am particularly interested in holism because of its focus on health care. Sudden death is a major health care issue, and can result in ill health as we have already discussed. One of the issues for Otto (1975) was that all people seek health. Symptoms are an expression of need and motivate the person to seek help. Emphasis is also put on life style and life goals, when working with the belief system and the meaning of life as seen by the person. What the sudden death means at the immediate time and later is always a major issue.

Within the holistic framework each person is considered unique. Within this framework, we can offer opportunities to help individuals manage or cope with the event. Before we look at another approach to sudden death, that is, crisis intervention, let us consider the person and the five dimensions of holism. Again, these dimensions involve issues in the immediate and the long term.

Physical dimension

In identifying personal stresses people describe how they react to certain situations. Worry, for example, gives 'butterflies' or 'a knot in the stomach'. Others get a rapid heart beat or sweat or feel cold. The stress of a sudden death, can also alter our bodies, and this in turn leads to feelings about our body image. In considering the whole impact of a sudden death, people will ask

'What is happening to me?'
or
'What has happened to me?'

They will perceive changes, some of which are clearly changes of body image — changes in appearance, or structure, size and shape. People will describe themselves shrinking or carrying a heavy burden which bends them. Restlessness, fatigue, sleeplessness and vulnerability lead to feelings of physical weakness. Threats to body image are stressful because the ability to relate in meaningful ways to others often depends on our view of our image. Our concept of our self-esteem or worth is closely interwoven with our body image.

Emotional dimension

Stressors produce emotions that generate physiological responses. How we view our coping capacity is often related to the intensity of our feelings or emotions. We all experience responses, for example, laughing, crying, fear, trust, being full of hope and strength. The more unhealthy responses of hurt, guilt, resentment, and helplessness cause us problems.

Absolute emotional health or illness is not something I know about. Emotional health is a process that evolves from emotional needs being met and a willingness to recognise and accept feelings, and perhaps use the energy generated.

Emotional health has close links with acceptance of oneself and harmony with that self. On the emotional spectrum we have to respond to change in ways that are either healthy or unhealthy. The intensity and duration of the emotions depend on where we are on that continuum, on our ability to satisfy our needs and experience, and to handle our feelings.

Intellectual dimension

The problem about the complex process of sensation or perception is that it employs the central nervous system. How this is functioning will depend on its state of health, which needs to be good to be efficient. Memory, learning, cognitive and expressive functions are necessary components of our intellectual dimension. Someone who is healthy will function in these areas more effectively than someone who is not. Recent and past events, and our memory of them, will help us to give current events meaning, and to understand them and even increase our ability to rationalise and cope with an event.

Defects of memory can affect our ability to conceptualise relationships. In the immediate impact of sudden death, and in the long term, perplexity and work concerning its meaning, much thought and concentration will be needed, e.g., an elderly lady suffering from recent memory loss or forgetfulness whose husband has died suddenly will have difficulty understanding the sequence of events around the death. This can cause her untold distress in trying to understand what happened around the event and involve a protracted counselling process for a carer attempting to clarify the details. Her need to examine the details is no less than anyone else's but will frustrate her and make her angry. Losing flow of thought through cognitive difficulties will cause untold problems in managing the death in the long term.

Difficulties for the old and confused, and people with mental illness and handicap, are specific examples of problems in this dimension. Healthy individuals need to be capable of using expressive function to express ideas and feelings. Ill health may prevent this. So a stressor in the intellectual dimension may be any problem that prevents receptive function, memory, learning, expressive or cognitive functioning.

Social dimension

Many events in individual's lives can contribute to social stress. Responses to social stress are determined by cultural values, past experiences in similar conditions, and our ability to cope with and understand the system. Relationships with support and nurturing may be found in our family network or we may have to seek them from other areas, such as work or close friends. Our position or social class within the system may give us strength or stature, or a role.

Social isolation or poverty, unemployment, marital or family difficulties may cause us problems if we have depended on these particular social dimensions for support. If we do not develop other social support systems when we are confronted with stress within our familiar system, we may not cope.

Social interaction, which is the basis of social relationships, can give us the right kind of stimulation. It prevents our isolation and stimulates thought and growth. However, too much interaction is a violation of our space and an infringement on our lives.

Much of the social dimension relates to our role. This may

be apparent when the social structure makes conflicting or impossible demands on us, perhaps demands that conflict with our value system or roles that are ambiguous. Some roles conflict with each other and some, because of lack of preparation or training, make us feel incompetent. A full use of our personal or professional resources results in a good utilisation of our role.

Some roles are temporary, others are imposed on us. In sudden death, this may mean all the aforementioned changes in the social dimension plus changes in sexual role and identity. The social dimension of sudden death requires a high level of adaptation and this produces severe stress.

Spiritual dimension

When people have to give a lot of attention and time to sorting out conflict that does not fit in with their belief system, the conflict then becomes very stressful. The inability to meet spiritual needs adequately, because of the conflict, leaves them in a kind of vacuum. This challenge to the individual's beliefs attacks values and the individual is left in an unclear and ambiguous life position.

Our philosophy on life may have cleared up or clarified our goals and values, leaving us free to follow our chosen path or direction. In turn, this decisive response will have confirmed our commitment to the chosen philosophy. Sudden death may question all this. Sudden death may indicate we got it wrong — we have failed because we did not reach the required standard. The wish to undo wrongs, to relive lives, expressions of shame and remorse, may as suddenly as the death become painfully apparent.

Spiritually healthy people have found reasons that give meaning to their existence: perhaps religion, or a relationship with nature and the universe. Some people have non-spiritual goals, such as money. Whatever the source of this meaning it gives them a sense of hope and the ability to overcome adversity. Lack of purpose and life without meaning leads to despair, feelings of being useless or abandoned.

In these periods of intense suffering people question the meaning of life and doubt their ability to overcome adversity. They question the value of the belief system they have or had.

Eventually these feelings can lead to withdrawal and an over-whelming feeling of not being able to invest any more energy in seeking answers. They are stuck with the outcome and have a sense of resignation to suffering. At the time of sudden death, much time and energy has to be spent on these very issues.

To review the holistic philosophy — each person is multi-dimensional. The five dimensions — physical, emotional, intellectual, social and spiritual — are in a continuing interaction with each other. The physical dimension involves everything that interacts with the body from without and within. The physiological and affective states, including motor mechanisms and the feelings that are involved, are included in the second area, the emotional dimension. The intellectual dimension covers receptive function, memory, learning and cognition. How we express this is also a function of the intellectual dimension. The social dimension involves social interaction and relationships as well as aspects of culture and the social systems. The fifth and last is the spiritual dimension. This explores how people develop their understanding of the meaning of life, and how this will transcend or overcome various life difficulties.

These five major concepts are generally accepted as the introduction and basis of holistic philosophy. I use them as an introduction to exploring responses to sudden death because our care should encompass looking into the immediate and long-term needs in these dimensions. They may offer a structured way of examining all components of the loss and prevent 'blinkered' focus, identifying the areas that are being avoided.

The important thing to remember is that they do not present definite answers to aim at, again identifying the holistic philosophy as one which attributes individuals with the ultimate responsibility for what they will do with the insights gained from looking at each dimension. This focus of control is very important to people who have lost control or become 'out of control'.

This framework may be useful in looking at areas of personal responsibility; the individual who has lost someone, who is suddenly bereaved, regains active participation and contributes to his own health status. I accept that some readers will find it difficult to assign health status to the response to sudden death. It may be that, for them, ill health is only recognised in the context of the medical model needing treatment from a medical practitioner with a passive participant. This is not the idea, and re-reading the basic principles will confirm that.

PEOPLE IN CRISIS

There are people in crisis in all areas of our work and with all types of conditions. Whilst some critical nursing areas, such as the Accident and Emergency Department, will be more likely to witness crisis, it is important to remember that we may come across a person in crisis in any setting. The fear produced by attending an immunisation clinic, or the implications of why this immunisation is needed, can be enough to trigger a major emotional upheaval whilst the parents of a young child with severe multiple injuries and with a poor prognosis face a catastrophe. A comparison of the two incidents may cause us to be judgemental about the participants; we may feel that the two cannot be compared, and yet the response to each incident may be a crisis.

Both incidents merit the same attention, the same commitment, the same non-value judgement. This is not easy, and our own family, class, culture and experience may not be at all useful to us in our evaluation of the event.

As we progress through this section, and through all our work, we will discover a great deal about our attitudes, beliefs, and value systems. If we allow ourselves to confront these or to be confronted by them, it will be to our advantage.

It is also important to begin with the concept of the person as indicated in the heading. The transition to the role of patient can be a de-humanising and therefore traumatic experience and it may in fact be the difficulties resulting from encountering a patient, rather than a person, that trigger off a crisis.

Different individuals will feel differently about being a patient, or client, some experiencing extremes of comfort or discomfort. It may be a totally new experience, it may be something witnessed in another member of the family, or it may have been experienced before. Two important factors in any resulting crisis are whether the experience is new or replayed and how it is perceived in that person's life.

These different reactions, and how they may result in a crisis, lead on to how our care of the client has evolved over the past few years.

The idea that clients can separate and present different parts of themselves to different people is obviously fraught with difficulty. Whilst we may not be experts at everything (and there will always be a focus of expertise) insight into the whole person is necessary. Some of the frustrations and difficulties of gaining a rapport with the patient will be removed if we have some skills in crisis intervention. The complexities and enormity of some clients' problems may be so daunting that we cannot even begin to help them cope with them. Crisis intervention will make some of these bigger problems manageable by helping to begin, and finding a focus in which to work.

With this in mind, I would like to consider using crisis intervention as an approach to the care of those involved with a sudden death.

What is crisis?

The Chinese interpretation of the word crisis describes it as an opportunity for change and personal development. This opportunity for growth and forward movement is certainly an entity, but the potential to damage, overwhelm and incapacitate is also present. Crisis may produce panic measures, and it is the panic aspect that ties in with our Western perspective of crisis.

We cannot say that some difficult events will inevitably lead to crisis. How we respond to the life event, and how it is perceived, will determine whether the outcome is a crisis or not. Stress and crisis are different. A stressful event produces anxiety and tension. A crisis disturbs old established patterns of responding, it demands a different and often new response. Whilst a crisis may not necessarily be a disastrous event, it can disturb our equilibrium and produce disordered behaviour.

Types of crisis

Crises are usually divided into two types: the developmental crisis which is associated with life's milestones, and the coincidental crisis which is not linked to any specific time in life.

Some of our clients' crises may be compounded by fitting into both categories. A 20-year-old woman, for example, may, within a month of her marriage, suffer the death of her husband in a road traffic accident. A developmental crisis, her marriage, is compounded by a coincidental crisis, the accident, which has the potential to throw her life into disarray. We cannot treat her loss, and the emotionally painful experience of the loss, without discussing the distress of all this happening within a month of her marriage.

Whilst this example identifies clearly the two types of crisis, others may not be so easily seen; we need to keep a sense of awareness of where the client may be on the developmental scale of life's milestones, in order to recognise the implications of a sudden death.

It may be useful if we place our client's loss somewhere along his life milestone graph (Fig. 1.1), noting the stage he is at, or may be heading towards or leaving. It could help us to consider where he may be in this area of his development and may, on further discussion with him, remove assumptions we have made about him.

Some of the coincidental crises, such as redundancy, divorce or separation produce a loss of status and security. Again, if these are marked along the line of life's developmental crises, their overwhelming nature will be perceived.

Phases of crisis

Caplan (1964), a world authority on crisis and the skills required to intervene, describes the four phases of crisis which indicate the intensity of the crisis and the individual's response to it. It is necessary to have some insight into which phase of crisis the client has arrived at because this alters the strategies we use in our care, and increases meaningful interaction.

A person may leave the crisis at any of the four phases (see Fig. 1.3) as he gains some access to resources within himself

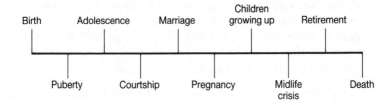

Figure 1.1 Life's milestones.

or elsewhere. This may involve his looking at alternatives and making choices, and this is where crisis counselling is valuable in enabling him to do this. There are three paths we can help him follow in order to gain access to the resources (Fig. 1.2).

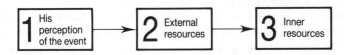

Figure 1.2 Three routes to explore when attempting to cope with crisis.

1. **His perception of the event** involves facing the reality of the event by asking him to describe the event and what it means to him, in terms of his plans, his hopes, his aspirations. How the event changes his life, the present and the future need to be discussed. The client's realistic appraisal of the event is important. Its impact and the likelihood of producing disorder are very apparent at this stage. The client will usually mention that self-esteem is damaged; what we mean by self-esteem will be examined in more detail later.

2. **External resources** available to help him cope with this event, and their whereabouts, are the second factor to work with. The disordered activity resulting from the impact of the event is often a very real factor in preventing a client thinking logically about sources of strength, comfort and support, and may actually prevent him from locating them. The first resources we head towards are usually family and

friends, or other people close to the client and on intimate terms with him. The person in crisis knows of his need of them but the disarray and distress produce fear that he will not reach them.

This may be expressed clearly as:

'Please help me find my brother, he will help me, he will know what to do.'

This expectation of the help to be received may will be initially unrealistic but as time progresses, and with help, more order will replace disorder.

The external resources may be other disciplines, caring agencies and organisations or self-help groups. It is important to be aware of local resources and the types of help available.

3. **The inner resources** of the client are what he can locate within himself to cope with this difficulty. This is not suggesting he will have the answer to his problems but that he should be helped to locate his strengths and vulnerabilities. The overwhelming feeling at a time of crisis is that any forward movement is impossible; the client is rendered impotent and this increases his distress. The fear produced by being immobilised is tremendously powerful; it can make one feel totally weak, or can produce panic measures.

Locating inner strengths and feelings can produce activity and movement forward, and potency or effectiveness. This feels good and it suggests some advance towards management of the problem. It is important for the client's self-esteem that he can ask himself the questions 'What can I do about this?' and can begin to look at answers and alteratives within himself.

The theory is, that if we can help the client to look at and work positively with these three aspects of the stressful event:

His perception of the event
External resources
Inner resources

a crisis may be averted. If denial of the meaning or the reality of the event is paramount, then the first area will have a strong negative content. If external resources are poor or not available, then the second area will produce negative results. The client's inability to locate resources, strengths or insights within himself will make exploration of the third area a non-productive exercise.

One or two negative responses to these three areas are likely to take the client into a life crisis. As described earlier, there are four fairly clear phases of crisis (Fig. 1.3), and which

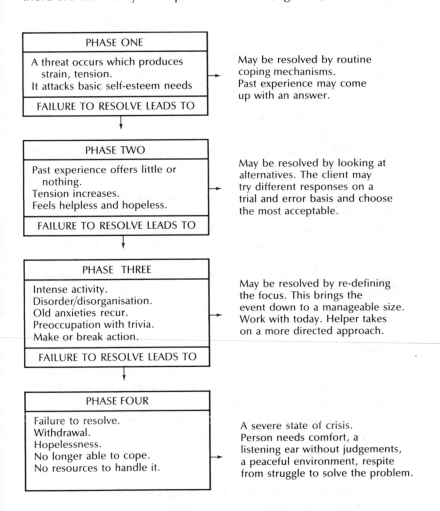

Figure 1.3 The phases of crisis.

of these phases the client is in, will determine the focus of our work with him.

The ability to recognise the client's position within the crisis process determines whether we facilitate a self-directed search for answers, or a more structured or directed approach. Failure to help the client achieve answers to his problems may produce a crisis for the carer. This can be distressing for people like nurses, who generally work towards clear or predictable outcomes.

A client's failure to find a way of working with his problems may be due to his refusing to acknowledge or explore the three areas previously mentioned, and it may be necessary to return to these areas. He may not be motivated towards a resolution in any case. We must be aware that we do not control outcomes and cannot always achieve success, whatever this means to each client. The ultimate success or outcome of our intervention lies with the client, and not with us.

You will encounter problems if you try to seek a quick conclusion to your crisis intervention. A sense of the real value of this work will help with your concern about your time commitment. Your initiative in helping someone to begin work on his crisis is important. The helper is in a unique position in that her role allows a degree of intimacy with the client which is not open to many others, and previously unspoken thoughts may be revealed by him at this time. You will, at these moments, gain insights into the many powerful emotional difficulties that could prevent complete recovery and will require the concentrated, motivated effort of the client.

Status

A sudden death can instantly or more insidiously attack a person's status. By status I mean the position or standing in society which governs the respect or rights people receive. Their status may give them a role or a place, somewhere they belong. If this is suddenly removed it leaves them vulnerable or seeking a new status:

'Where do I stand now?'
'Does this relate to what I thought I had?'
'This is like starting all over again.'

Some people describe having to make a completely new start or an about turn. Image and status can be closely bound together. Return to the life's milestones graph and place your client in the appropriate place along this line. We have discussed how this may indicate a developmental crisis; it may also highlight a threat to the client's status. It may, for example, indicate a shift towards retirement or a mother's children growing up and leaving home, or the end of a woman's sexually reproductive period. All these changes may demand a new role and a change in status.

THE DETERMINANTS OF GRIEF

In his 1975 study, Parkes identified determinants or predictors of grief. These are factors in a death that determine difficulties in working towards a satisfactory outcome. (You may note my avoidance of the word 'resolution,' which is often used in crisis work. One question I have often been asked is:

'Is grief ever resolved?'

It would perhaps be more appropriate to say that one works — or struggles! — towards living with this loss.

The determinants of grief from the Harvard Study are listed below:

```
1. Mode of death
2. Nature of the attachment
3. Who was the person?
4. Historical antecedants
5. Personality variables
6. Social variables
```

Box 1.2 Determinants of grief.

I would like to make some observations about these determinants from my own experience of counselling people who have suffered a sudden death. Over my years in acute psychiatry, counselling and critical care nursing I have discovered the value in having these determinants identified.

They identify focuses of difficulty which become recurring issues in the counselling. If they are borne in mind when you share your client's account of the loss, you will not fail to be aware of the part these components play in his reaction to the crisis.

They may be dealt with quickly or trivialised because the client feels intense pain when considering them. You may need to return to the painful area later and an awareness of the determinants helps you to do this.

1. Mode of death

If the death was from 'natural causes' such as an illness, even if it was sudden, it is likely to cause fewer problems than traumatic death. Death by injury, death which damages the body, is more likely to be thought of as causing suffering and as being an injustice.

Most people will ask whether the deceased will have suffered or known anything about the act or process of dying. It will be more difficult to blame others if the death was due to illness, but they may blame themselves in this situation for not having the foresight to call a doctor sooner, or an ambulance. The professional ability or resources of individuals in the Health Service may be blamed. Much more time and effort will be needed to explore the issues around this. We cannot blandly absolve them from any responsibility. They will need to do this for themselves.

Death by road traffic accident, or accident at work or at home, can cause anger and a sense of injustice far greater than the natural sudden death. This is made even worse when monetary compensation is an issue — this usually falls short in that it somehow devalues the deceased.

The verdict of the Coroner's Court or findings of the Fatal Accident Inquiry is often discussed at length, as is the question of whether the deceased was entirely blameless in relation to his own death. If the deceased was not to blame, something or some person is usually felt to be responsible. The area of responsibility may be even wider — if a person or organisation was not to blame then culture or society may be blamed. In some extremes, civilisation or mankind is blamed and the bereaved person may isolate himself from society.

This type of condemnation results in an even greater loss because of its resulting isolation.

John's parents believed that the importance attached locally to traffic and commuters resulted in or contributed to John's death. Commuters parked on both sides of the road on every working day: there was no car park despite local pressure for one. As a result, the road was narrow and its curve also caused problems, particularly for heavy goods vehicles.

John and his friend died instantly when John's motorbike was struck by a lorry. They were thrown into a wall and died of multiple injuries. There was evidence that they had been driving too fast, although this was disputed. What was not disputed by any witnesses, including the lorry driver, was that the lorry had had to cross the centre of the road because of parked vehicles.

The official verdict was accidental death. Recommendations were made about parking restrictions. John's parents were pleased about this but who allowed it in the first place? Why does everyone need a car? Perhaps we should sell ours to make the point that we are destroying the environment with all these cars.

Over a period of months, much of their grief was worked through well. The anger and its power were diminished. Their resentment of the city's traffic policy, and how they were surrounded by it, were a constant reminder of their belief that society values people less than cars.

Eventually they moved house which resulted in further losses. Despite this, living in the country gave them some tranquillity and less ammunition for their anger and frustration about the destructive effects of traffic.

When considering the mode of death, the location becomes an integral part of the grief. Was the deceased on home ground or in a strange place? The pain will be greater if he was far away from home. He was all alone when he died. No person around will have known him and this underlines a recurring theme that he was someone special, a big, important part of their lives. Away, he was a stranger, no-one knew him, he was anonymous, alone. His real identity, the person he was, was not apparent.

The fact that many families are now scattered throughout the world presents an added dimension to grief. This is particularly difficult if friends and neighbours did not know the deceased.

Mary received a telegram to say her brother in Australia had died suddenly. He was her only brother. He had emigrated 20 years previously, and when Mary's neighbour came to comfort her she attempted to reduce the enormity of the loss by reference to this: 'Well, never mind, you lost him a long time ago, in a sense. You couldn't be close after all this time.'

Mary kept her sadness to herself after that. Her guilt at not making the effort to visit him would remain hers. No-one here knew him, they had no sense of his love, his warmth, his happy personality.

The carers, friends, neighbours and family may be at a real disadvantage in having no sense of who the person was. It can reduce their ability to understand and empathise.

One mode of death that produces some tremendous difficulties is suicide. The process of grieving somehow becomes very complicated both emotionally and intellectually. The bereaved are not only sorting out their own loss but going through mental exercises about how the victim might have emerged from his difficulty if he had remained alive. They may even come up with some answers that would have prevented the suicide, and that of course is the potential for some profound guilt.

In counselling, the one thing really valued is a chance to express some powerful, ambivalent feelings. I would, without hesitation, suggest that people closely touched by suicide will be in need of some counselling.

2. The nature of the attachment

There is clearly plenty here that can be explored and below I identify briefly some of the issues. The strengths of the relationship, what its loss represents, and the security or aspects of safety that they gained from the relationship, are two areas useful to explore because they will highlight vulnerability.

One feeling recurs time and time again in this and any crisis, and that is ambivalence; the strength of this will, in retrospect, give rise to much heart ache and soul searching. Where there was ambivalence in the living relationship, it will certainly occur at the death and in the long term. The difficulty lies in the strong sense of its being inappropriate in grief — much time can be spent in trying to enable the expression of ambivalence.

3. Who was the person?

Who the deceased was in relation to the bereaved person sounds like asking the obvious, but this must be ascertained. The deceased's position in the hierarchy of the family is not necessarily a clue to the enormity of the loss and we must not make assumptions.

I can still remember talking to and trying to comfort the lover of a middle-aged man, whilst his wife sat in a room a few doors away saying she was now free to get on with her own life. Not only is the family relationship an issue, but how would you feel if your husband died at the home of his lover?

4. Historical antecedents

A previous life crisis, particularly a sudden death, will present as a major factor in coping. If I have experienced a previous life crisis with a good or reasonable outcome, then in theory this should help me. I will have programmed into my head something that identifies difficulty but removes or diminishes some fear about the outcome. This may be useful, provided I can be in touch with the previously programmed material; I have discussed earlier in this chapter why this might not be possible (see The Intellectual Dimension, p. 18).

If the previous outcome was one of pain and suffering, the present problems are compounded. Previously unresolved loss, or previous failure to confront loss, may result in its re-emergence causing difficulty for the helper in establishing the focus of the loss.

Other recent life changes, or crises, or recent depressive illness will result in more difficulty in handling the loss. Lots of energy and resources used up in tackling these will have left the person drained or depleted of resources.

5. Personality variables

From my own counselling experience, I have found that personality affects the search for a healthy resolution to grief. Problems in the long term can be caused by negative factors, though the reverse can also be true in that positive coping with the immediate grief does not guarantee a lack of long-term problems. The personality that allows self-actualisation, a feeling of some control over one's own life, and sees problems as a challenge would seem to be the one most likely to recover.

Raphael (1984) writes that although no specific risk factors have been demonstrated it has been suggested that certain personal characteristics lead to a risk of poor outcome. These again were ambivalence and dependent and clinging relationships.

Earlier personal experience of grief, especially childhood loss of parent/s, contributes to vulnerability. I have witnessed this vulnerability re-emerging in my workshops, and it would seem that this childhood loss is diminished only with difficulty.

The key variables in influencing an outcome in this area appear to combine personality with pre-existing relationships of dependence, something akin to the chicken and egg story.

6. Social variables

Some loss alienates and isolates, other loss produces gain. The gain may be freedom to leave a group or community or restrictions, for example those of a sexist relationship. If the person left was, or felt they were, an extension of the deceased and fed from their social network, the enormity of the loss becomes apparent.

Some religions and cultures will feed and nurture the bereaved, and shower them with offers of help and validation of their worth. In the UK there are diverse examples of community response to death. Clear confrontation of it, or avoidance, are reactions in communities not too far apart. How our social and cultural backgrounds influence our caring role will be explored in more detail later.

Whilst Christianity and other religions are thought to be a help and support in sudden death, it may be perceived otherwise:

Miriam was 28 years of age when her 6-month-old baby died suddenly. She has one other child, aged 2½ years, and she is married to a solicitor. She is Jewish and has a large extended family living far and near. Her baby died quickly from overwhelming infection, at home in his cot. Miriam found him but was quickly removed from him.

Many people came and cried with her, and cared for her and her husband and the other child. Food and drink were brought and the housework done. Whatever she asked for she got.

As is the custom, her baby boy was buried within 24 hours. Within a few days some of the activity had petered out but she described herself as being well cared for.

Years later Miriam feels as though something was not completed. She resents the 'indecent haste' that her religion inflicted upon her. She wanted to be with her dead baby and hold him, to have a chance to say goodbye. To actualise the loss in this way she feels would have helped her towards a more satisfactory coping state. She is resentful and angry that the rites of her religion prevented a more gentle separation that was somehow part of and under her control.

That day, events happened very quickly and she feels she was imposed upon, not only by the death but by the ritual that should have given her comfort in distress. It was like some intense activity that left her with nothing.

She now feels that if there were a next time, she would have to choose between her apparent emotional needs and her religion.

In looking at these determinants of grief, at crisis intervention and at the five dimensions of the person, I have identified three ways of working with sudden death. These are the results to date of my search to find meaningful ways of caring for the victims of sudden death. To establish some rapport in this situation is difficult because of the bizarre and intense aspects we encounter — aspects of madness, chaos and disorders.

These three approaches will, I believe, help to put some order where there is disorder, and restore meaning and insight where there seems to be madness. I know insights are not enough and that some of the quality of life needs to be restored, and there are many other approaches.

My search for other approaches is not over. Those discussed above highlight not only what may be useful, but also many difficulties. The immediate difficulties are explored in the next chapter.

REFERENCES

Caplan G 1964 Principles of preventive psychiatry. Basic Books, New York
Glick I O, Weiss R S, Parkes C M 1974 The first year of bereavement. John Wiley, New York
Holmes T H, Rahe R H 1967 The social readjustment rating scale. Journal of Psychosomatic Research 11: 213
Lindemann F 1944 Symptomatology and management of acute grief. American Journal of Psychiatry 101: 141–149
Lundin T 1984 Morbidity following sudden and unexpected bereavement. British Journal of Psychiatry 144: 84–88
Otto H 1975 Wholistic therapy. In: Harper R (ed) The new psychotherapies. Prentice Hall, New Jersey
Parkes C M 1975 Bereavement — studies of grief in adult life, 2nd edn. Penguin, Harmondsworth
Peppers L G, Knapp R J 1980 Motherhood and mourning. Praeger, New York
Raphael B 1980 Primary prevention — fact or fiction? Australian and New Zealand Journal of Psychiatry 14: 163–174
Raphael B 1984 The anatomy of bereavement: a handbook for the caring professions. Hutchinson, London
Shanfield S B, Benjamin G A H, Swain B J 1986 Parents' responses to the death of adult children from accidents and cancer: a comparison. American Journal of Psychiatry 141(9): 1092–1094
Wordon J W 1983 Grief counselling and grief therapy. Tavistock, London

2

The immediate needs of the family

In this chapter, I will deal with some of the clearly stated or implicit needs. Again I must explain my reason for approaching the care in this way. Just because some needs are clearly requested or apparent does not mean we have the resources, the ability or the will to deal with them. Many of the immediate needs will be obvious to us — some of the significance of this will be explored as well as some of the difficulties. How this aspect of the care was perceived later, or its implications in the long term, will be examined in the next chapter, following through my approach in dealing first with the difficulties that we all know about. Later, I will discuss the way this was reflected upon in the long term by families or friends, and how we may improve on this care.

One of our misconceptions about the relatives of sudden death victims concerned the recollection of details. Each relative was asked to describe events in the hospital on the day the loved one died. The amount of detail given was surprising. People describe very accurately the layout of the room to which they were taken, details of the picture on the wall, and walking through the department (the department is complicated even to those who work there). The nurse or doctor who cared for them was described in detail, even to the colour of their eyes.

It would appear that during this period of threat and distress we have a heightened or more acute perception of events. It is important that this is emphasised to prevent the attitude that what we do or say does not matter too much because they will later suppress this painful event. The idea that relatives will block out painful memories is common among people who work in hospital critical care areas, perhaps because it helps them to deal with not engaging with the family for very long periods. It could be a way of dealing with our deficiencies in our care of the families.

The fact is that families describe very accurately what happened to them, and in great detail. Whilst I must describe behaviour associated with certain emotional responses in this chapter, this will be explored in greater detail in the chapter on training.

Relatives who have not travelled in the ambulance will arrive later and be placed by reception staff in the relatives' room. In contacting them we will try and ensure they ask for a named nurse upon arrival.

THE RELATIVES' ROOM

One relative said he wanted to return and place a notice above the door stating 'The Good News Room'. This gives some indication of the strength of feeling about what occurs within these walls. The majority of relatives seen appreciated the following facilities offered within or near the room:

— a telephone, with access to dial nationally
— a wash basin, hot and cold water, and towel
— chairs and coffee table
— privacy
— drinks
— access to toilets.

The criticisms of the room were about its size and its oppressive nature. The room has no outside walls and therefore no windows. This produced panic and fear if relatives were left alone. They wondered what was going on outside the walls and were unsure as to whether they could leave the room or not. They described the lighting as dull and one lady insisted she was left in the room with no light at all. The nature of what is said in this room is dark and oppressive and I am sure no-one was left in the room with no light at all. As a result of this feedback the size of the room used has doubled, and it has lights, and a window which looks out onto a corridor where activity is apparent. The window has curtains to prevent others witnessing the distress within.

To be able to see activity outside the room helps to some degree with the tremendous feelings of isolation and the fear this produces. It is important to be able to re-evaluate how the surroundings can have a strong negative effect on an already distressing situation. The privacy and yet accessibility were both factors commented upon favourably.

THE VIGIL

The person who cares for relatives within a hospital emergency department or other areas is usually a nurse, although some hospitals use a social worker or chaplain. Where crisis intervention is practised, or hospitals have liaison psychiatric departments, psychiatric nurses with special training in bereavement or crisis counselling may be used. The nurse doing this work can also answer questions about the physical and emergency care, and the feelings associated with this.

It is difficult to separate discussion about the whole question of resuscitation and the imminent or possible loss from the feelings associated with it. For this reason I think a nurse is the best person for the job in the immediate care. The nurse is likely to be able to liaise between the resuscitation room and the relatives more comfortably than most others, and will also have some knowledge about the emergency treatment.

The initial care of relatives who were not present when the emergency occurred will concern the identity of the patient. This may involve finding a suitable moment during the resuscitation to take the relatives to look at the patient in the resuscitation room. If the patient is going to the operating theatre quickly, it is important to establish positive identification prior to this. This will prevent relatives having to sit with uncertainty for a long time. Even if you positively know the identity, relatives may stay with the unreality until they have personally set eyes on the patient.

This uncertainty, if a factor, will produce more difficult behaviour for the carer who will witness relatives expressing opposite ideas about the reality. Questions about injustice and guilt, and other profound and difficult issues, may be discussed:

> 'It cannot be him, we are so happy, everything is going so well for us now.'
>
> 'Please tell me it is not true. He was due to be somewhere else at that time'
>
> 'I know it is him. It's not fair. Bad people live, why is this happening to us?'
>
> 'How can you believe in God when this happens?'
>
> 'Don't say any more. You are making a terrible mistake'.

The issues raised may produce a very real discomfort in carers, confronting them with issues they have previously avoided. It is difficult to be in the role of carer and supporter and yet not have the answers.

The nature of the injuries or illness may mean a prolonged period with the relatives before a patient dies or is pronounced dead. Serious head injuries, for example, may require brain scans, insertion of intracranial pressure measuring devices and neurosurgery. At some time during the process of care, the patient may die. News of procedures to be performed may give hope that is seized upon with unrealistic expectations.The patient going for insertion of a pacemaker may not survive and suddenly, all hopes are dashed.

This produces feelings that are very obviously opposites. The time spent with relatives, whilst many resuscitation procedures were being carried out, was measured for the 100 deaths in our study.

Table 2.1 Survey of 100 sudden deaths — time spent by nurse with relatives of patient who subsequently died.

Time spent	%
0–1 hour	27
1–2 hours	46
Over 2 hours	27
	100

You will see from the results shown in Table 2.1 that the time with the relatives on many occasions was 2 hours or more. Two hours is a long time to witness and share another person's extremes of anguish and distress.

LOSS OF AUTONOMY

One issue with very pertinent implications in this part of the study was the overwhelming feeling of loss of autonomy experienced by the relatives. It brings in the issue of advocacy, some clearly sexist material and the difficulties for the nurse in having to deal with these issues. An awareness and sensitivity to these crucial matters will facilitate something very important in the long term, and the way these issues are handled in the immediate term will also be of particular importance in beginning that process we call grief.

It is necessary that most people have some feeling of control over their lives. Plans will be made, hopes and expectations will give us some feeling of comfort and movement. Suddenly, this is all thrown into chaos and confusion, pain and hurt:

Mrs Jones sat rigid in the relatives' room awaiting news of her son's condition. Paul was 8 years old, her only child. He had been hit by a bus when crossing the road on the way home from school. His friend had run home in panic to give the news of Paul's accident. A neighbour had confirmed that it was Paul, and an ambulance had taken him to the Accident and Emergency Department.

The nurse told Mrs Jones that Paul's condition was critical, and asked if she wanted anyone to join her at the hospital. As her husband was away working, she asked for her mother and mother-in-law. Her words were almost inaudible. Now and again, she asked fearfully if there was any news.

When her mother and mother-in-law arrived, the nurse left for the resuscitation room to seek an update on Paul's condition. The team was talking of abandoning further efforts as there was no sign of life. The nurse was grateful that Paul did not look too bad as she returned to the relatives' room. Paul's mother looked so fragile and the nurse was frightened that further information would cause her to break.

When she was told there was no improvement, and the outlook was poor, she just whispered 'Thank you.'

It was an hour after her arrival that a doctor joined Mrs Jones, the nurse and the family. Everyone knew the gravity of what he was going to say and yet hoped they would be wrong.

'Your son Paul has just died. I am very sorry.'

Paul's grandmothers wept openly and held Mrs Jones, distressed that their comfort evoked little or no response. The doctor carefully explained what measures had been taken to restore life and how it was to no avail. They thanked him for his efforts and Mrs Jones asked him flatly if Paul had suffered. She was confidently assured that he had not.

When the doctor left the room there was silence for a while and then Paul's mother asked, 'Can I see him?'

The nurse's relief at this first reaction was mixed with anxiety at the distress Mrs Jones would feel.

'Yes, of course you can,' she said.

Her mother quickly became very agitated: 'You must not do that. It is best to remember him as he was.'

Her mother-in-law confirmed this: 'It won't do you any good — let's just go home.'

'I would like to see him,' Paul's mother whispered.

The words did not convey the longing in her heart just to have another glimpse of his face.

'Just take it from me,' her mother said, 'You must not. You don't know about these things.' Her voice was desperate. She just wanted to get away.

'Why prolong the agony? We'll take her home,' they said to the nurse.

The calm and sadness were rudely interrupted by a voice not previously heard. It was strong and determined: 'I want to see my little boy. Take me to him.'

The nurse led her away.

When she returned to her mother and mother-in-law she was weeping and could not be consoled. Her cry was one of torment and questions. 'Why? Why?'

'We told you not to' they said.

When Mrs Jones was seen 10 months later she clearly remembered the struggle to see her son. She described how she nearly lost the battle, and how she had always believed in her mother's authority. Her struggle to speak, and wondering if she was being heard, was crystal clear to her. She was powerless and at the mercy of all around her, and her fate was to lose.

She is not clear where she found the strength from to state firmly what she wanted. What is clear is that the nurse quickly used the opportunity to take her to see her son. For this, she was so very grateful. She wanted to be with him and quickly, and was glad she could see him just where he was when he died. Her memory is of him lying on the resuscitation table draped in a white sheet, and seeing the shape of his genitals under the sheet. When she saw this and his washed, white face she just knew it was her little boy. She held his hand, wept and said goodbye to him.

Now, 10 months later, she clearly knows the value of this time and how she was nearly denied it. The loss is borne alone, however, as Paul's death is a taboo subject with her husband. Her comfort comes from her joys with Paul and her goodbye. Her secret of the value of the goodbye is simple to her:

Since her childhood she has believed that anyone injured in this way would be squashed flat. To carry this image around with her would have been torment and misery. She knows, as I do, that for most people, reality is far more acceptable than fantasy. Fantasies are bizarre and cruel, and can be uncontrollable. Reality gave her comfort. Reality confronted her with the starkness of death, but it was still preferable to her long-held belief of flattened people.

For me, this was the beginning of confirmation that the truth will set people free of some of the pain. For the nurses, this process of taking people to touch, talk to and sit with the deceased is painful and time-consuming. The confirmation of its value is important to us. Many others spoke of the value and ambivalent feelings of spending time with the deceased. Not one person in our study had any negative feelings about spending time with the dead person. Many had regrets at not doing so and for some the thoughts they had to conjure up as to how the deceased looked were cruel and tormenting.

The relatives in this situation need someone to act as advocate for them. This will be useful in the long term but they are often powerless to ask for it themselves. They are unaware of what is allowed and what the rules of the organisation are. They might have lived with someone for 20 years but cannot be sure if they can ask to be with them and for how long. Another thought they have is that we have too much to do for the living without spending too long on the dead. One elderly lady said:

'I was so grateful when the nurse said there may be things you want to say to your husband. I did not know, you see, if you were allowed to or if they would think I was barmy talking to someone dead. It made it natural, it made it all right. She held his hand when we went in to him and she said I could. You do not know what you can do, what is allowed. It was very special for me having that time together. He was my husband after all, but we need to be told what we can do.'

Once through the doors of the institution the patient is no longer entirely the family's or the individual's. They relinquish part of him to the organisation and are reluctant to state their own needs and do not know what boundaries are imposed upon their needs and behaviour. We are needed to facilitate what will be useful and positive. An insight into the constraint that people perceive is necessary, but it is not enough. We have to state clearly what is allowed in fairly explicit terms:

'You can hold his hand if you want to.'
'Feel free to talk if you have things to say.'
'I am sure you want to say goodbye.'

These examples of how individual autonomy is compromised by the organisation are closely linked to the issue of viewing the body. There is another issue in the immediate care where the bereaved need an advocate:

SEXISM

One of my greatest difficulties has been coping with the many young widows and trying to help them with their immediate needs. Male sexist behaviour and responses are an issue even in death. On many occasions, young wives have a need to hold and weep and share last moments together with husbands. It seems to me to be a perfectly natural thing to do. However, older male relatives arrive, or male friends of the husband, and tell them they must go home and it would be better if they did not do it. This profoundly disadvantaged person, rendered weak and ineffective with no control over her life, usually acceeds to this person of strength and knowledge.

Do men do this because they need to be seen to be taking control? Will the distress produced by her contact with the body be too difficult to control or witness? I am sure that the men's underlying need is to look after themselves or to be seen to take positive action in a very difficult situation. Once they have taken this stance it is difficult to convince them otherwise. To invite contact with the dead person appears to be imposing pain and distress on someone already very distressed. The easy way out is to let this person take over.

The ritual of a short vigil and goodbyes is a healthy and positive start to leaving someone behind. The bereaved need our help to begin this journey. The prevention of contact with the deceased creates problems for mothers who have experienced Sudden Infant Death Syndrome or other infant and child deaths. This over-protection, though well meaning, can have long-lasting implications.

It must be re-emphasised that not one person in our study had regrets at seeing and spending time with the deceased. We must be aware of the sexist issue and then we can help the bereaved to verbalise and focus on needs that are difficult for them to stay with.

The ritual of time with the body may be linked to this, to staff avoiding this painful area and also to the resources and time it demands. Many staff describe opposition to a vigil from mortuary staff, and many describe struggles with relatives of the bereaved. This confrontation with the reality of the death will be the real difficulty for many because of our Western culture. Whatever the underlying cause, we must use the insights we have received in our feedback from the bereaved, to help relatives with their immediate needs.

INFORMATION

Whilst the loss is the real focus of the event, there is a definite need for clear, understandable information. This may make some sense in a situation that is outside the realms of understanding, as there is a strong need to add order to a chaotic situation and to remove some of the perplexity. Families valued honest direct information about the sequence of events and from people who did not skirt around the real issues. This makes sense of the structure of the crisis intervention model and dealing with the first issue of realistic perception of the event. This information giving has the underlying effect of being loaded with confrontation.

BREAKING BAD NEWS

The first contact doctors will have with the relatives in most cases is to break the bad news. It is felt that final confirmation of death must come from the doctor's own mouth although there are occasions when it is the nurse who gives the final confirmation. For the doctor, it is usually a transaction with strangers at a critical time in the strangers' lives. The nurse will, by this stage, have established some rapport with the relatives and be present when they are given the news.

We asked relatives how they felt about the way the news was given. Many of the relatives felt the doctors performed very badly when they spent the usual brief time with the relatives.

Some of the immediate anger I have witnessed has been when the doctor has taken a long time to give them the awful news. Some have asked various questions about the patient's past medical history and have then given the news. Others have gone into a preamble prior to the final words and this has produced anger. The main criticism was not about this but

Table 2.2 Survey of 100 sudden deaths — time spent by doctors with relatives, after giving confirmation of the death.

Time spent	%
0–5 minutes	51
6–15 minutes	23
15 minutes or over	8
Doctor not used at all	18
	100

about basic communication skills. One woman described the doctor as:

'Performing like a bus conductor, swaying on both legs with one hand on the door post and looking into the distance.'

Most negative remarks were about the doctor not sitting down and being on the same level when the news was delivered. It was interesting to note how many commented on poor eye contact. Some relatives were unable to leave the ramifications of how the news was given, and it proved to be a difficulty in moving into the reality of the loss.

The use of euphemisms is to be avoided. Words such as dead or died are unequivocal. The idea of often-used phrases:

— He has passed on.
— He has slipped away.
— We have lost her.

may be well meaning but are open to misinterpretation or may feed someone's denial. One man told us:

'When the doctor came in and said I am afraid we have lost her, I thought what a damned fool. How could they allow a woman who is so sick to leave the hospital? You see, my wife was always a bit wayward and if someone said something she did not want to hear she would just walk out.

I remember saying what do you mean? How could you just let her walk out? He looked embarrassed, and said she is dead. I remember being angry and saying:

"Well, why didn't you say so?"'

PROPERTY

One woman, when visited 10 months later, asked the researcher to help her remove from the bottom of the wardrobe a bag of clothes given to her on the day of the death. It was something not bargained for, and appeared symbolic in relation to the stage this lady had reached in her grieving process. Some relatives complained that they were not asked to take away clothing, and others said they were, despite the fact that it may have been cut or bloodstained. It became apparent that some nurses felt the family should be given the opportunity to take away the clothing, whilst other families were protected from this. Despite the fact that presentable white cardboard carrier bags were available, many people were given clothes in the easily accessible white plastic bag. This took on a great significance:

'I went in with a wife and came out with a dustbin liner of clothes.'
'They just stuffed his clothes into a dustbin bag without folding them properly.'

It was easy for people to find hidden meanings in this, and some felt it reflected the sort of care people received. It is just another example of how some issue, distant from the main focus, can take on enormous significance.

I personally feel that to arrive at the hospital with a person and to leave, after the death, with a few possessions, confronts the bereaved with the reality of that person having been left behind. For this reason I prefer it to be part of the immediate care and not postponed until later. Nurses, when told of this response, insisted that they do explain when clothing has been cut from the patient to gain access for resuscitation. But perhaps the nurses do not make this clear because, in a sense, it does deal with a difficult or distasteful aspect of the death.

DOCUMENTS

Along with this handing over of the property, relatives are given a booklet with information about what do after a death (DHSS). We also give a list of information produced by the hospital on how to register the death and obtain a death certificate. This shift to some very practical aspects of the loss may, and often does, produce a marked change in emotional response. There is a controlling nature to this confrontation and the need is seen to 'get on with the practical details.' A response at this stage often refers to practicalities:

'I will have to carry on somehow.'

The other interesting response at this stage is the way the loss can be depersonalised. This may be expressed as:

'Of course this is a common occurrence for you.' or
'People die every day and others have to get on with it.'

This emphasis moves it to a national or global problem.
Another common response when there has been a move to this area of thought is the attention being turned on you, the nurse:

'How do you cope with doing this all the time?'
'What an awful job you have.'

The assumption that may then be made, which may suggest a way of us coping with it, is:

'Well, I suppose it's just another death for you.' or
'This is just part of the job, is it?'

The shift from its personal meaning, and the need to put it into some other perspective, may be a move that proves difficult for the carer. It may be welcomed as a shift from the personal pain, but the move can mean entering into difficult areas such as the meaning of sudden death. The idea that this little scenario is being played out all over the world in many varying locations, is one whose significance they can ponder on. The problem for the carer is that they may be questioned on its meaning and then feel uncomfortable at not having the answers:

'How do others cope with this?'
'Why now?'
'Is there some message for me somewhere in all of this?'

At this stage the family may request the services of a chaplain or other religious support, or you may offer this to them. In sudden death, it is not at all unusual for the response to be anger, and you must be prepared for this. It is important that the likelihood of such a response does not prevent you making the offer. For people with a religious belief it is important they are given the opportunity to express this.

THE IMMEDIATE RESPONSE

Depending on culture and race the immediate expression of grief can be noisy and emotional, or quiet and apparently showing little emotion. However the lack of obvious response does not mean that the relatives are not grieving. The initial reaction is often one of disbelief, numbness and possibly denial; after a few minutes when this has worn off, they may then begin to cry or respond with anxiety, guilt or anger. In an attempt to understand this event they may begin to question what happened, reviewing it several times, and demonstrating a great need to understand what led to this event.

As events are reviewed, the sad and painful outcome may produce strong feelings of distress. Staff need to be patient and to be prepared to allow this to happen more than once. The need for answers is paramount. 'What did he die of?' is the question everyone will ask. Tentative ideas about this may be discussed and explored. This inevitably leads to a discussion or to the realisation that more conclusive evidence will be available at post-mortem, and the need for this.

The search for answers then shifts back to the awful reality of the death, with the focus on the dead body. The idea of the post-mortem and the mechanics of this often produce anger and a return to intense emotional feelings. This pattern of mental activity — searching for answers, trying to make sense of something senseless and then experiencing uncontrollable feelings — frequently becomes apparent, and we as carers are working with and responding to that 'see-saw' pattern of to and fro, up and down. They will apologise for this and need to know they are not abnormal and will need reassuring on this point.

The other question they will ask you is:

'Is this really happening?'

or, of themselves:

'Am I dreaming?'

An immediate need, then, will be to sort out the reality of death. The role of the carer is vital in re-affirming this aspect of the whole event.

HELP TO FIND RESOURCES IN THE IMMEDIATE

Some extremely simple tasks become very difficult or complicated. Information habitually familiar to them will become difficult to locate. Family, friends or significant others, though geographically near, will seem far away. Those who are far away will cause the helplessness and frustration to intensify. Even people familiar with telephone directories will ask you to find someone's number, because they cannot understand its sequence.

It is not at all uncommon for people not to be able to use the telephone or dial a number. Which persons are significant in their lives, and how you can arrange for them to join you, is an important issue. It often requires painstaking discussion to elicit where these people are. It is important in a large and busy Emergency Department that relatives and friends are able to ask for a named member of staff on arrival. To arrive distressed and find that reception staff do not know who you are puts both staff and relatives in a difficult position. It also suggests that this most significant of events is not demanding our priority.

Some relatives will negotiate with you prior to the arrival of others as to whether you or they should give them the bad news. I feel it is important at this stage that they have to impart this information. You have to begin to encourage this, reluctant though you may be.

ARRIVAL OF THE RELATIVES

The arrival of other relatives and friends will produce some intense distress and a feeling for the carer of beginning it all again. Again, the events leading to the death and why it happened will be reviewed, perhaps more than once. You may use this opportunity to evaluate how the person who was at the hospital from the start perceives and relates to the event. It is useful to allow them to relate it to people who join them, as it will again confront them and give them an opportunity to review the death.

When you hear this you could well hear other things being clarified. Other family and friends arriving may give further opportunity to spend time with the deceased. The moment when all meet, and this time of being with the deceased, is often when all the pain and anguish becomes apparent. The family may, at this stage, spend some time together alone. Do not assume they want to. Check it out.

ADVOCACY

The most significant person in the deceased's life may now be at risk from being swamped with care. I am not sure why this so obviously happens at this stage. People recalled the problems it caused them as will be discussed later. If a person has been alone with the immediate grief, it is as if this must be compensated for and the people arriving must take over responsibility for them. They begin to answer for them, they make decisions for them, they direct them in any way possible.

One of the roles of the carer in this immediate situation is to protect the bereaved from this, and it will be resisted by the additional people if all that they can give in the situation is to be seen to be in control. It will be more of an issue where the arriving relative is a male caring for a female. In a life crisis such as this the immediate pain and chaos are unbearable. Attempts to replace it with some order and control may involve a loss of autonomy for the person closest to the deceased. This issue is described in the earlier case study (p. 41).

If you wonder why these aspects are being repeated or reinforced, it is because that is how it is in reality. It is also an indication of how time consuming or complex the whole care may seem when families are large and when many other people arrive. If that suggests it can be too difficult or time consuming to undertake, we need to return to the question why do it at all? The whole story here in this book will, hopefully, tell you that. The message that remains important and should be uppermost in our minds about this immediate care is the same. The bereaved will never again have the chance to work through this most difficult time in the immediate term unless you give them the space and time to. It can be an opportunity which has the power and the potential to begin the process of grieving and which should not be lost.

The advocacy role of the carer is an important concept to stay with. The notion of advocacy is best described as when individuals need help and support to pursue their own needs and interests. It will help them to find a voice when they have difficulty speaking for themselves. It will often deal with a conflict of interests such as the difficulties of the relatives overriding the needs of the bereaved.

Relatives or friends often take you aside or clearly have a need to speak to you alone. They are at a loss as to how they will care for or cope with the distress of the bereaved, and they will often want direction on this. Some questions are about definite issues:

'Should I take her home with me?'

Others are more difficult with no clear answer:

'What can I say to her about this?'

The distress or helplessness of the friend or relative often leaves you feeling as anxious for them as for the bereaved. Be prepared to give relatives some time and opportunity to talk about their anxiety if this is possible.

The task is now becoming even more difficult. Needs of individuals are increasingly diverse and confrontation situations can easily arise.

ABSENT AT THE TIME OF DEATH

Because most sudden deaths will require vigorous attempts to resuscitate the patient, most relatives will not be present at the time of death. Many will not be present in the hospital, and others will be kept waiting in a different room. The majority will ask, when death is confirmed:

'Did he suffer?'
'Did he know what was happening?'
'Did he say anything?'

Some people can place the focus more precisely on the issue most important to them and say:

'Did he ask or say anything about me?'

Strong ambivalence is expressed at not being present at the time of death — a great need to have been there and an equally great need to run in the opposite direction. When this ambivalence has settled, many will regret or feel guilt at not having been present.

We can give clear information and should not avoid answering questions. Often we will be confirming that the patient was unconscious and had no awareness of what was happening around him. At other times we will be informing them that strong analgesic drugs were given to deal with the pain. Supplementary information about the nature of these drugs confirms this, and can alleviate further distress. We may further state:

'The drug was a powerful narcotic, like morphine.'

Most people have heard of morphine and understand its useful properties.

Despite all these reassurances there is a difficulty for the people who are left. Issues such as why they did not get to the person on time, and their helplessness in trying to facilitate this, can become prolonged difficulties. Because of the clear value for most people of being present at the time of death, we must not forget waiting relatives when attempts at resuscitation have failed. Some patients will continue to have a heartbeat for a short time after attempts have ceased. The relatives can be brought to the patient to spend a short time with them before they die.

The separation of family from patient has been identified as causing difficult and often disruptive aggression in emergency departments (Wright 1985). Work in a USA hospital explored whether relatives should be present whilst resuscitation was taking place (Doyle et al 1987). It was found that relatives may wish to be with family members who may be dying, even though resuscitation efforts are being made. Seventy people who participated in the study were taken to the resuscitation room, accompanied by a member of staff, who explained what was happening. None of the participants interfered with the resuscitation efforts.

The participants were later contacted, and 47 responded. Forty four (94%) of these respondents who had been present during the resuscitation believed they would feel able to participate again. The conclusion of that study was that the presence of the relatives during resuscitation led to the perception that they had been able to help the person undergoing resuscitation. This in turn was helpful to the grieving process. They saw no reason for continuation of policies that exclude family members from the resuscitation room.

When efforts are discontinued and there is still a heartbeat it is important to disconnect the patient from the monitor, otherwise relatives watch the monitor and it can cause problems of concentration in the interaction with the patient. There is also the added difficulty of them witnessing the trace 'going flat,' and this producing alarm and distress. It will also be much kinder to the relatives to have removed intubation tubes and intravenous lines. If it is not possible for relatives to be present at time of death most appreciate seeing the deceased as soon as possible afterwards.

SEDATION

The issue of whether someone should be sedated when suffering the acute distress of grief after a sudden death will probably become less of a problem. My feeling is that this request is less common than it was 10 years ago. Some will check it out by asking:

'Is it still thought to be harmful to sedate someone in this situation?'

The most grief-stricken person, in the immediate throes of a sudden death, rarely asks for sedation for themselves. It is usually for someone close to them and if the person they are requesting it for overhears, he usually rejects the idea vehemently. The common thought at the time is, of course, do they want sedation for the relative's pain or to prevent distress to themselves on witnessing the pain.

There is no doubt that most people who have been sedated or have begun to take tranquillisers know of the problems that this has caused them. Many of the people I have seen for bereavement counselling have regretted the recourse to chemical help for their grief. It is to be avoided if at all possible.

SUDDEN INFANT DEATH SYNDROME

There are some obvious and apparent needs of bereaved parents where there has been a 'cot death'; but difficulty with the reality of the death, and confronting the death, will be a problem for both the parents and for us. We will feel less certain about what we should do and then ambivalence will compound this difficulty.

Again I will look at what immediate needs appear to arise, and in the next chapter share with parents the benefit of hindsight. Many parents will have the benefit of hindsight within 24 hours.

An apparently healthy baby is put to sleep in a cot or pram. Occasionally the baby has some minor symptoms. These may be a snuffly nose, or perhaps he did not take as much feed as he normally would. When next looked at the baby is dead. It is slightly more common in boys than in girls, and more frequent in winter months. In the UK about one baby in every 500 live births dies suddenly and unexpectedly. In many parts of the world it is the most common cause of death in the age group of 1 month to 1 year.

When later examined by a pathologist, a small number of these babies revealed a previously unsuspected abnormality or an overwhelming infection. In the majority of cases, however, death is difficult or impossible to explain. In the absence of any known cause these deaths will be registered as Sudden Infant Death Syndrome.

On present knowledge of this syndrome the death cannot be foreseen by parents or doctors. Most of the babies will die silently in their sleep or if not asleep rapidly become unconscious and die. There is no indication they suffer distress or pain. Those found face down or covered with a blanket may cause the parents to think they suffocated and that they are to blame. External suffocation, however, is not the cause of Sudden Infant Death Syndrome.

Sometimes vomit is found around the mouth or on the bedclothes. This will lead to the conclusion that the baby choked on his vomit or his last feed. Many parents bemoan the fact that they did not spend enough time with the baby or 'getting his wind up' after a feed. The presence of vomit occurs during or after death and is not in itself a cause of death in these babies.

When a normal baby dies there just has to be an answer. It must be explained. The reason I have gone through all the previous information is because these are usually the aspects questioned about. These question may in the immediate situation be repeated time and time again. The search for an answer inevitably leads parents to ask who is to blame. Parents can blame themselves, the doctor, the health visitor, the baby sitter, and frequently God.

Over half of Sudden Infant Death Syndrome babies arrive in Emergency Departments. The apparently overwhelming grief and distress may cause the ambulance personnel to bring the baby to hospital alone. They have a need to remove the pain (the dead baby) from the parents, or they may not have had time to wait for the parents in their urgency to resuscitate the baby. Parents may not have been able to leave other children who are at home.

When they ring the hospital later, both parents should be invited to come to the hospital as soon as possible. This may be resisted if someone knows the baby is dead. A typical response may be:

'Is there any point in bringing the mother?'
'Can you just confirm the baby is dead.'

Many times, both parents will arrive and when death has been confirmed, will want to see and hold the baby. The role of the Coroner's Officer* (policeman) will need to be explained. It is important that as much information as possible is imparted, to deal with their helplessness and perplexity. A paediatrician will give this information more validity.

You will need to explain that other relatives, such as grandparents, will want to see the baby and they must feel free to bring them along. The offer of open access to the dead baby prior to post-mortem is important. How this was perceived by parents is re-evaluated in hindsight in the next chapter.

*England and Wales only

It is important that the parents are not left alone unless they request it, and that they have the opportunity to review the whole of the event prior to departure. The arrival of the other significant people in their lives will allow them to re-live the events. This process, often called 'the obsessional review' will be a major part of the ongoing grieving process.

If the mother is breastfeeding, she will need immediate advice on the suppression of lactation.

Written information to take away with them, on what we know about SIDS and on obtaining further help, is available from the Foundation for the Study of Infant Deaths. The address of the organisation is in the appendix on page 175.

This is perhaps the right place to remind hospital staff that all clothing removed from the baby should be placed in separate bags for collection by the Coroner's Officer. This includes soiled clothing and nappies. Nothing should be discarded or destroyed. Although the baby may have been placed in a clean gown, you may wish to offer the parents the facility of returning with the child's own clothes and maybe a favourite toy.

IDENTIFICATION

For legal reasons, many sudden death victims need a formal identification in the presence of a police officer. This always includes cot deaths and other trauma victims. This may be possible where relatives go to sit with the deceased and the police officer discreetly withdraws after the initial contact. He will later obtain a statement to the effect that they identified the deceased in his presence. If you forget that this is necessary, the parents have to return to the hospital or mortuary and repeat the procedure. This needs explaining to relatives. Many, I know, prefer to keep this more formal procedure separate from their own time with the deceased, and separate from their own goodbyes.

LEAVING THE HOSPITAL OR PLACE OF DEATH

Prior to their leaving, you may want to check that the relatives have all property or items of jewellery that were with the deceased. It will be a time to confirm they know what procedures to follow next. It is important to check that they know how to contact you to clarify what may have happened or for more information.

No-one should be allowed to leave alone if at all possible. In the past 12 years I have only known one man insist on this. Help in arranging transport, or obtaining a taxi, should be given.

The act of leaving presents great difficulty for most people; once the initial feeling of wanting to take flight has diminished, people often feel the opposite. It is hard to leave their loved one behind. This is often expressed in a comment such as:

'Take care of him, please.'

The final act, in dealing with the immediate needs of the relatives, is helping them to leave. We can acknowledge their difficulty:

'I know it is hard for you to leave him here.'

They will be confronted with the separation and loss in this part of the procedure. It is often the trigger for a re-emergence of overt distress. It is an opportunity for you, the carer, to say how sorry you are that you could not do more to help them. It may be the final confirmation of your awareness and distress at the awful outcome for them. People appear to value this being acknowledged.

The whole process of the immediate care is time consuming and emotionally very demanding on the carer. How we pick up the pieces for ourselves and the organisation will be discussed later.

To re-iterate, this chapter has looked at apparent and implicit component parts of the immediate care of relatives where there has been a sudden death. Because in the immediate term the grief-stricken person is put at a disadvantage, because he does not know what to ask for, because he has been left weak, impotent and sometimes speechless, we must meet unspoken needs.

Some needs we know about, because words are not always necessary for communication. But with hindsight, people were able to say what they had needed and whether these needs were met.

REFERENCES

DHSS What to do after a death.

Doyle, C J, Post H, Burney R E, Maino J, Keefe M, Rhee K J 1987 Family participation during resuscitation: an option. Annals of Emergency Medicine 16: 6

Wright B 1985 Hostility in accident and emergency departments. Nursing Mirror 161(14): 42-44

3

The value in reviewing the events of 'that day'

When the relatives were visited later, they were asked to describe the care given to them in the immediate situation. This care had some link with the grieving process and the link can be identified in what the relatives told us.

The process of reliving that day, and describing the events, also had some interesting repercussions. Some of the insights gained by people, and by ourselves in retrospect, will be described. Certain kinds of sudden death were identified as resulting in more pain and long-term difficulties.

Before we look at the responses of these bereaved people, it will be useful to review what others have said about the grieving process. We shall take the opportunity to examine how sudden death might differ from death where there is opportunity for anticipatory grief, as discussed earlier.

THE PROCESS OF GRIEVING

Many people, writing about the subject of grief, have discussed the stages or processes through which the bereaved pass. Kübler-Ross (1969) , for example, describes five stages:

- denial
- anger

- bargaining
- depression
- acceptance

but this does not mean we should always expect the bereaved to clearly and obviously pass through each phase.

Wordon (1983) prefers to use the word *mourning* to indicate the process which occurs after loss, and he refers to grief as the personal experience of the loss. He describes these phases as passive states which differ from what he calls the tasks of mourning. Tasks imply some input or work, and suggest some activity on the part of the bereaved. This ability to have some input into what others call the process, Wordon sees as being particularly valuable. It also returns us to the problem of some of our bereaved who feel a loss of control over their lives. Wordon's views may therefore have some particular implications for them.

Of course, Freud's famous paper (1917) on mourning and melancholia also talks of grief work. The implications of both these ideas are that the mourner needs to take action and do something rather than wait for something to happen.

The idea that outsiders can, by intervention, do something to assist in this work is partly what this book is about, but it would also seem to me that we have to allow certain feelings to emerge. The acceptance of these feelings and their validity, and allowing the bereaved to confront and explore them, may be the mixture of passivity and activity that is necessary. Many of the people I have seen have worked at the problem night and day, and need to give looking for answers themselves a break to allow what seem to be the most important issues to be identified. It may be that they need someone to help them do this.

Parkes (1975) describes alarm, searching, mitigation, anger and guilt. He ends with gaining a new identity. This process seems to be one of activity and is doubtless hard work. The guilt may overwhelm the bereaved with sadness, and may even immobilise them.

So the process, or stages of grief, will probably consist of both working through certain tasks and allowing certain feelings or phases to be experienced. There is validity in both approaches.

It is interesting that Cook & Phillips (1988) in discussing the stages or phases, name one of them 'resolution of grief'. In my workshops, when I talk of the final stage as being re-solution, many people invariably feel the word to be inappropriate. They immediately see resolution as finally bringing the grief to an end, and as being a definite termin-ation of a difficulty.

The same anxiety is expressed by clients in bereavement counselling, in that the end of the counselling is seen as in-dicating that the deceased has finally been put to rest or allowed to fade into the distance. The bereaved do not want this, they want to remain close to the deceased, and so may resist that part of the process which some call resolution.

According to the Shorter Oxford English Dictionary (1983), resolution is defined as:

1. The process of resolving or reducing a non-material thing into simpler form, or of converting it into some other thing or form.
2. The answering of a question; the solving of a doubt or difficulty.
3. The removal of a doubt on some point from a person's mind. Certainty, conviction, positive knowledge, resulting in determination, firmness or steadiness of purpose.

These all appear to be admirable places to arrive at, or suitable states of mind to begin change with. Resolution, then, is perhaps a word that describes the end of the process or stages of grief.

Bowlby (1981) reinforces the idea of passing through these phases before mourning is finally resolved. He points out that there are overlaps between the various phases and that they are seldom distinct.

Kübler-Ross (1975) describes how this process can help the bereaved to emerge strengthened and enriched by the ex-perience. She describes death as providing a key to the meaning of human existence and offering a chance to come to terms with death as part of human development.

So if people are given the opportunity to grieve, then they should sooner or later progress to feeling confident and posi-tive about their future life, and will again experience some enjoyment or fulfilment.

I feel that the way they begin this process is of paramount

importance. The ways in which people in our study were helped to start grieving indicate the paths that carers can follow in order to facilitate grief at a sudden death.

Jane was sitting alone in the relatives' room when I walked in. It would be better to describe her as crouching with her arms wrapped round herself. She rubbed and squeezed her arms and body, and the anguish was apparent on her face.
'He is dead, isn't he?'
Fifteen minutes before, her only baby son had arrived in an ambulance, lifeless. The resuscitation measures had just been abandoned. There was clearly little hope on arrival, and he appeared to have been dead for some time. After this was established, and as we were discussing the baby as being a victim of 'cot death', I was interrupted. 'His mother has arrived,' were the words that quickly shifted our thoughts to the distress of his poor mother.
John, her husband, was driving down separately, and Jane had sat in the front of the ambulance as it sped through the streets, siren wailing and blue light flashing.
Jane's whole posture and overwhelming sadness were visibly apparent. There was no hope, no request for him to be spared, no denial of the awful reality. She knew. My nod of the head and hoarse 'Yes' confirmed what she least wanted to know. She cried and held my hand, and inattentively stroked my arm, her thoughts elsewhere.
'You won't leave me, will you? Where is John?'
She quickly filled me in on Adam's short life, assuring me he was loved and wanted, and how in the 12 weeks he was alive he had begun to thrive and have a personality of his own. One idea had been that he might be a musician. What a great gift, she said, to make people happy with music.
'I must have done something really wicked to deserve this. How stupid not to notice he might be ill or sickening for something.'
The reassurances that this happens without warning or symptoms, and how we believed he was the victim of Sudden Infant Death Syndrome afforded little apparent consolation.
The paediatrician arrived, and told Jane how our immediate efforts to find signs of life had produced nothing, confirming that when Jane found Adam at home he had been dead. He

went on to tell her what we knew about Sudden Infant Death Syndrome, and told her how he would send for both Jane and her husband in 5 weeks' time to discuss it again.

When the doctor left we suddenly realised that John had not arrived, and soon afterwards a phone call from a neighbouring hospital informed us that he had arrived there. In his turmoil, Jane's big strong man had rushed to the wrong place.

'That's not like him,' Jane said. 'Quiet, strong and well organised. Poor John, he didn't know what to do with me or himself.'

John's guilt at getting to the wrong hospital and not being present to comfort Jane was soon verbalised on his arrival. He held her whilst she cried loudly and painfully. (Such a cry that once you have heard it you know what it means.) I explained to them that I would arrange for them to see Adam, and how they would both have much to say and reflect upon together with him. Jane said at once:

'Yes, take me to him now.'

I left them together, explaining I would need to check that everything was ready for them to see Adam. As I was leaving the room, John turned to a very fragile looking Jane, sat her on his knee and held her to him.

Adam was, by now, in a clean baby gown and wrapped in a blanket. The staff had taken a great deal of pride in seeing that he looked just right for his parents and someone had put a single flower in his hand.

Jane, well supported by John, entered the room and immediately both of them began to cry loudly. Jane lifted Adam up and cradled him in her arms and her anger and distress were painful.

'Why have you left me and hurt me in this way?' she asked.

'Please come back, come back,'

'Wake him up, please', she begged me.

'I wish I could,' were all the words I could muster, and John looked at me pleadingly:

'Please help her, please.'

He looked around helplessly, and this strong grown man began to shake and thump the palm of his hand in his frustration and helplessness. He was so used to putting things right for his wife. Jane was by now walking up and down, holding Adam tightly to her.

'Can we take him home, John, and just bury him in the garden?'

'No, Jane you can not', John replied. 'Tell her not to say that.'

Her thoughts were elsewhere and John began to shake and cry. Jane was now sitting, holding her baby.

'I am sorry,' John said, 'please let me go outside, I need some air.'

I left the room with him. He stood shaking and looked ready to explode with the grief.

'You want to be strong for Jane,' I said. 'But who would be a Dad at times like this. Dads feel pain, feel grief and feel helpless. Who looks after you?'

He held on to me and wept bitterly, and I held him. No words were spoken for at least 5 minutes and then he put into words exactly what was happening.

'I need so much to hold on to you and for you to hold on to me.'

There was the acknowledgement that he had both these needs and he was giving himself permission to have both.

We returned to the room and Jane was sitting quietly, rocking to and fro more peacefully. I explained that Adam was in our nightdress and that they might feel better if he was wearing his 'best' clothes or something of his own. He may have a favourite toy that they would prefer him to have close to him.

We began to talk of grandparents, aunts and uncles, close friends, and the need to inform them. Jane and John were both assured that all were free to come and see Adam in the Chapel of Rest if they wished. Jane particularly was advised that she and John were free to return day and night within the first few days, and was warned gently that she might wake in the night and wonder where he was. It was important that at times like these she should know where she could come and see him.

Whilst the last thing in the world she wanted was confirmation of where he was, this is, in my experience, preferable to not being able to see him. The hours of the night are long and lonely, and using this period to hold the baby and reflect can offer some comfort. Jane said she knew she would have to take me up on the offer.

After I had spent some time explaining the involvement of the Coroner and the need for a post-mortem, they prepared to leave. Literature from the Foundation for the Study of Infant Deaths was handed to them, with written details of my name and telephone number. As they left, both said they might possibly need to return and talk, and John said, half smiling:
'I may need you to cry with again.'

Both did return, on several occasions. Over the next 2 or 3 days, they called and sat and held Adam in the hospital chapel. His favourite toy elephant was brought, his bright red suit and his only lace-up shoes, that Jane felt so good about putting on his feet.

His grandparents, aunts and uncles came, some together, some alone. In Jane's periods alone with Adam, she was sometimes angry and remonstrated with him for leaving her, and then was angry with herself for loving him too much. One morning, when John said he knew how she felt, she protested loudly that he had never been Adam's mother.

Both decided on the 4th day that they would not visit after the post-mortem. They sat alone with Adam and said final goodbyes. As Jane handed him back to me that night she said
'I know this is it now. He cannot be with me any longer.'

They quickly said goodbye and left. As they walked out I thought of all we had achieved together, and yet knew this was only the beginning.

Jane and John's experience was one of the 100 sudden deaths in our Leeds study where the bereaved did not respond to our request to take part in the study. The feedback I received was over a year later, when Jane asked to see me. She described much love and support from John and their family and friends, and her involvement in a group for 'cot-death mothers'. She valued the sharing of experiences and the support this group gave her.

She returned to give me two messages. One was to say they were slowly emerging from this 'and from time to time you must have a need to know this.' How right she was! Secondly she wanted to say how much she had valued that immediate care, and that she now realised how much work she had done at the time.

The word 'work' was hers. She described her confrontation

with death, with its awful reality. She then recalled her unhurried opportunity to reflect on Adam's short life in the presence of his death. This confrontation with death's reality, and her realistic perception of the event, clearly ties in with one of the three components of crisis intervention that we have to work with.

The action Jane found most useful was, in many respects, what was the most painful. She recalled the moment she handed the baby back to me, having arrived at the decision not to see his body again. She told me how important it was to finally feel able to do that:

> 'I did so much work in those 3 days to be able to arrive at that moment.'

She described how she had come realise this from her encounters with other mothers who had experienced cot deaths. Some had not been given the opportunity to work in this way in the immediate situation, or were prevented from doing so by themselves or other well-meaning people. She described herself and the others who had responded and worked in the immediate situation as being months and maybe years ahead in the process of grieving.

It was clear to Jane that the immediate input in the hospital had begun that process we call grief, and had allowed her to begin to re-emerge from the distress it caused. She had done this sooner than the others who were not given the same opportunities or freedom to encounter death; their ambivalent feelings and distress, although painful, were then encountered again and again, and the difficulties of denial were less apparent.

Jane confirmed for me what many other parents of 'cot death' babies have since told me. At the immediate time of the loss, and on subsequent days, the bereaved parents must be given one or more key workers, and several hours, to talk through the loss and to encounter the dead baby as frequently as they wish.

The opportunity to deal with the feelings of anger as well as grief, and talk through all the details of the death, is tremendously important. Time to reflect on the life of the baby, and on the nature of the relationship with parents and others, is the beginning of a recurrent need to review the details of the death.

This detailed review of what happened at the time of the death was something commented upon by all who responded to our request to take part in the survey.

THE REVIEW OF THE DAY OF THE DEATH

We wrote to 100 people recorded as next of kin where there had been a sudden death. The typed letter was short and to the point, and a stamped addressed envelope was enclosed. The letter was signed by me and came from the department where the death had been confirmed, i.e. the Accident and Emergency Department.

The letter simply asked if we could visit them to discuss what happened to them at the hospital on the day their loved one had died. We stated that the purpose was to try to improve the care we gave to relatives when a sudden death had occurred.

A consent form was included with the letter, and we requested an address or telephone number at which they could be contacted. Permission was given to use the information for the purpose of the study.

I must emphasise at this point that any details which could identify individuals or families has been omitted. Although the case studies in this book are based on fact, some names and details have been altered to protect the identity of the people involved. Only one person expressed any anxiety about confidentiality and how the material would be used. People were very keen that it be used to help others in a similar situation.

The response rate was high despite the sensitive nature of the material. Table 3.1 gives details of this.

One of the conditional responses was 'Only if you do not bring medical students.'

Since looking at the returns and thinking about the people who had moved house, I have become aware that this change of house is an issue often discussed in my bereavement counselling. The question here is should we move quickly or wait until we have worked through the grieving process. People

Table 3.1 Survey of 100 sudden deaths — responses on being asked to discuss the sudden death.

Response	%
Signed response to agree to be seen	51
Letters returned by Post Office 'Gone Away'	4
Conditional response, e.g.	4
'Only without my husband'	
'Only with my husband'	
Objection or angry response	1
No response	40

are, of course, aware that the move may reflect an attempt to leave the pain behind.

Only one person in the study was seen at the hospital, and this was at her request. Since this study, and because we offer the facility for people to return and talk to us, many have returned. They are able to discuss the difficulty of walking through the doors into the department again, and returning to the room where their worst fears were confirmed. The opportunity to do this appears to satisfy some need to return to the pain and experience its distress but also to be able to disengage from it again. It also helps the process of retracing or reviewing the events.

Everyone seen for the review of events was seen by my colleague, Marjorie Ashdown. As I had been involved in the immediate care of many of the relatives, Marjorie was able to be a more objective listener. I also felt that it would be easier for the bereaved person to be more critical or negative about the department.

Before she carried out her visit, Marjorie reviewed the nurse's appraisal of the relative's emotional response, and the details of the circumstances of death; these had been elicited by me from the nurse within 24 hours of them caring for these relatives. The information obtained at this time included details of who, if anyone, was with the significant relative, and whether they spent time with the deceased. Whether property was taken away immediately, and the total time spent in the department, was also recorded and available to Marjorie.

The average time Marjorie spent listening to each person or persons was 3 hours. It is significant that, without exception, everyone said they had never related the whole story before.

This became important because the opportunity to review the whole history gave new insights, new meaning or understanding of the events, and removed some of the perplexity.

Despite the aim of the exercise being to review the events within the hospital, and this was explicitly stated, most people were unable to remain within these parameters when relating the events. The whole day has major significance, and ends with where and how they slept that night. I have since, in my bereavement counselling, been able to use the question:

'What happened to you on that day?'

Events and interactions both before and after the catastrophe become extremely important.

'I know now, after telling you all this, what I have not done. He never went to work without saying goodbye. It was just another day. I had piles of washing, I remember now. I will hang it out when he has gone to work, I thought.

We valued that time together in a morning. It sounds silly I know. It was really warm and I thought this is stupid, get it out and get it dry. I'm a very practical person, you see.

When I saw his car going out of the gate it annoyed me. He can't even just stop for a moment and say cheerio. I was thinking about him and waiting to say goodbye to him. It never even crossed his mind. Selfish thing, I thought. Typical of men. It sounds stupid now, doesn't it? I have just realised. We never even said goodbye.'

When this lady was called to the hospital, a caring neighbour who accompanied her advised her not to see him when she was told he had died of a heart attack.

'Better remember him as he was,' she said.

She never did get to say goodbye properly. Her review of the whole episode gave her the answer to what was unfinished. She went to the cemetery a week later to do what she now realised she had wanted to do for a long time, to say goodbye. She was also able to express her guilt at feeling annoyed with him as he left her. Once she got this out of the way, she progressed through the other stages of grieving.

Whilst all the issues may not be as clear cut as this one, the review of the whole episode deals with the frustration and perplexity of the sequence of events. The impact of the event produces chaos and disorder, and there is a great need to restore order. The review helps to do this.

Several people in our study contacted us again and asked if they could tell it to us all again. Although many of these bereaved people had loving, caring friends and relatives they had not told them the whole story. Listening to the review of events is not only time consuming, it can also be distressing, as can witnessing the grief of the bereaved person. I suspect they were diverted from it, or interrupted, before the story was completed because it was felt to be harmful to them.

For those working as bereavement counsellors it may be important that the first session is 2 hours long, to allow a complete review of the day's events. This will very often clarify some difficulty, and produce an immediate sense of resolving some issue or changing the focus. This makes a very important contribution to the beginning of counselling.

This obsessive review can also highlight any difficulty about the focus of the pain. People become fixed on some aspect of the event which appears trivial. This focus grows and becomes an irritation, yet they cannot disengage from it.

'When I collected Tom's clothing from the hospital, his jacket was not there. I later found it in the car. Why was he leaving the shop to go to the bank without his jacket on? It was not a very hot day. People must have thought it was odd when they saw him lying there collapsed with no jacket on. He looked smart with it on. If he had been wearing it as usual perhaps he would have been all right. When I picture him lying there without it, it seems all wrong. It is just not him. I just cannot understand why he was without it.'

We eventually progressed to a passer-by having begun cardiac massage and mouth to mouth in an attempt to resuscitate Tom. This led on to the sequence of events culminating in confirmation of his death. This shift of focus was painful and difficult, and led to the widow finally discussing his absence.

Her attempts to avoid this had resulted in her preoccupation with some less pertinent aspect. She spent many hours pondering how his death might have been prevented, and somehow the jacket became part of this. She was able, with help, to move on to how life would be for her, without Tom.

Clients are very often angry with themselves for the way some of these peripheral issues take on enormous dimensions.

The review of the event — a detailed look at the whole day, and how life was prior to and after the death — is time consuming and painful, but may well highlight some difficulty or perplexity previously unresolved. For both client and counsellor confronting the impact of the loss and beginning the process of separation will redefine many issues involved in the process of grieving.

THE VIGIL

The time of waiting between arrival at the hospital and being given the news of death varies considerably, depending on the cause of death. The difficulties in experiencing extremes of feelings and disordered behaviour, during this period, were described later as torment.

Table 3.2 Causes of death in our 100 sudden deaths.

Cause	No.
Medical, i.e. Cardiac arrest, subarachnoid haemorrhage etc.	63
Road traffic accident	12
*Suicide	7
Sports	2
Work accident	4
Home accident	3
Surgical emergency	1
Cot death	8

* This was atypical

If, for example, the cause of death was trauma, it is possible that prolonged measures of intervention, in the resuscitation room and then theatre, were undertaken before death occurred. Some patients with serious head injuries may have been transferred from another hospital and had a CT scan, prior to theatre. Some time during this evaluation and resuscitation process the patient may die.

Patients who arrive in cardiac arrest, having had a heart attack, are often dead prior to arrival at the hospital, and someone has to make the decision to cease resuscitating them.

The traumatic deaths were more likely to be younger people, and our time with the relatives was likely to be longer. The relatives of those who were traumatised by some outside force, such as a car or a piece of machinery, produce other problems. The deceased is more obviously a victim of someone else. If someone dies of a heart attack and it was felt he brought it on himself because he worked too hard, it may be more difficult to blame someone else.

For some relatives, then, the wait can be up to 2 hours. It may be an hour before they know whether their relative is going to live or die, and up to 1 hour in the hospital after they have died. The later chapter on what incapacitates the carer gives a more detailed breakdown of these times. The longer the experience of not knowing whether the patient would live, the greater the difficulty both at the time and later. The immediate ambivalent feelings were also a difficulty later:

'When waiting to hear if my husband had survived the accident I begged him not to leave me, just to get well. I even threatened him and said don't you dare die now. At the same time I told him I loved him and I could not have found a better husband.

The awful thing is he did die. I kept going over it all again, pleading with him saying come back, tell me it's all a dream, and then getting angry with him saying he had an absolute nerve to go when we had so much to do. Between this I told him I was sorry I had not told him enough that I loved him. It was so frustrating, going round this thing in this way all the time.

You must think I'm mad. I'm not, am I?'

There is obvious difficulty, then, in suddenly experiencing the question of will he live or die, as opposed to the statement 'He is dead.'

'They just said I am sorry he is dead. Just like that. The end. I got up and said, "Well, that's it then. Shall I go home? What do I do now?" There is no way you can argue with the fact that someone is just dead.'

Whilst some people may slip into denial, the clear fact of death leaves no room at the time for negotiating anything else. The statement is final. It is the end.

Even though the sudden death from a heart attack or other medical cause is a difficult death to come to terms with, sudden traumatic death is even more so. Obvious ambivalent feelings and disruptive distress and disorder were still apparent at both the 6 month and 10 month period of follow up. This group also described more disruption and difficulties in family relationships. The cot death and the suicide families also identified for us many issues to explore and clarify, and powerful difficulties in relationships.

People who became very disordered in their behaviour, or displayed marked ambivalence in the immediate time around the death, were showing signs of this later. At the time of the death, it would be more useful if we could more accurately predict who would be more likely to be at risk physically and emotionally from the loss in the early stages. Knowing who would need the most support would be very useful, particularly if this could be shown to prevent long-term damage and breakdown in relationships.

Although Chapter 1 has described how some deaths are likely to be more difficult to recover from, our feeling was that the traumatic, suicide and cot deaths left people with some very distressing problems. Most of the people referred to me in my capacity as a bereavement counsellor fit into these groups. Many of the issues reflect difficulties that were apparent in the hospital or at the time of the death, but were not worked with appropriately or easily.

It was also of interest that where people had exhibited a clear emotional response in the immediate situation, such as anger or denial, this was still an emotion they were continuing to work with or have difficulty with. It appeared that it was not only the immediately expressed emotional response which was a later issue, but also how it was responded to and worked with.

One lady, seen 6 months after her husband's death on the rugby field at 39 years of age, said:

'First of all can I apologise to you? You must think I was awful. I am not really that sort of person. When I saw him just

lying there dead that day, I was so mad. I said, "You bastard, you have left me to bring up three kids alone."

I actually hit him. He had been out enjoying himself and ended up dead. Do you know, I actually hit him on his chest. Tell that nurse I am sorry I embarrassed him. It's funny, because he said, "Don't worry about that. You have every right to be angry, left in the position you are in."

Later, when I felt angry, I did not feel bad about it. As the nurse said, "Who wouldn't with what's happened to you today."'

It was important to that lady that someone in the immediate situation was able to use that opportunity. Her guilt about her response could have been so destructive. Instead, she was able to acknowledge she had needs of her own. This is particularly difficult for women who are told:

'Take care of the kids.'
'Be strong for them.'
'His mother will need your help and support.'

In this case, despite being told all that, she was able to accept her guilt in a useful way and ask for things for herself.

PACTS PRIOR TO DEATH

Some couples or families will have discussed, prior to the death, how they would prefer the partner to respond or cope on the death of one of them and particularly who would 'go first' and what the implications of that might be. This is often discussed at the time of death.

'I should be grateful for her sake that it's her and not me to go now. She always said she wouldn't manage on her own and she wouldn't. For that reason, I should be thankful that this is how it is.'

He will also need to know at the time that it's difficult to sustain that thankfulness, and how difficult it will be to reconcile it with his grief and despair.

Some of the wishes imposed upon our loved ones regarding

death can result in some distressing and difficult problems and may damage the remaining partner. If this is raised at the time of death, we may be able to talk about the problem and its potentially damaging aspect.

'He always said I wasn't to grieve for him when he had gone. We had a long and happy life together. We had so much to be thankful for. All sorts of awful things happen to people, they get divorced or have affairs, or end up out of work. Well, nothing like that ever happened to us. He said that whoever went first we were just to think of the good times we had together, and be thankful that nothing terrible ever happened to us. He wouldn't have wanted to see me distressed like this.'

That sort of 'condition on how to respond to death' can be extremely powerful. To have to control one's grief, despair and sense of loss, because of a previously imposed wish, causes many problems. It is obviously done with the best of intentions, as no-one would like to visualise their loved ones grieving, and their hope for them would no doubt be that they would recover quickly. We need the process of grief to heal us and allow us to re-emerge from the power of our loss. To ask someone not to grieve is wrong. It is taking away their opportunity to recover.

I find it useful, when spending a longer period with someone at the time of death to ask:

'Did you ever discuss the possibility of this happening?'

This can give the opportunity to discuss last wishes and how they are not always useful. Some people will need permission not to adhere to them, and as we are sometimes seen as someone in authority we may be able to release them from a pact. If you are working with some long-term difficulty, it is essential that this issue is dealt with. It can so often be the key to facilitating the process of grieving

SUICIDE

For people bereaved by a suicide, 'who was to blame?' is the issue that either preoccupies them or is carefully avoided. The major assumption is that someone must be to blame. There is no doubt that the relatives we saw were extremely anxious about how the material would be used, and whether they were doing the right thing confronting the problem. It would appear that the issue is either taboo, or one that produces hostility and breakdown in relationships. They feel it is therefore best avoided, unless the blame can be apportioned to their satisfaction.

Evidence collected by Henley (1983) expressed the view that death by suicide results in a bereavement more devastating than any other form of death. In particular, the very negative social reactions towards surviving relatives and spouses have serious consequences. Lack of emotional support and practical assistance was a striking factor in Henley's study. She describes a massive avoidance of communication regarding the suicide.

My experience has been to remove the myth that there is a focus for the fault as soon as possible. It is just not that simple, and many factors influence the eventual outcome. We may even collude with the idea of finding the key, the answer to it all. If we have been influenced by a particular school of thought, our reaction may be coloured by that.

Freud (1917) described the death drive as inherent in all people, in a constant struggle with the will to live. This, he said, accounts for the ambivalence in suicidal people.

Durkheim (1951) offers a sociological approach on suicide, saying it is related to the socio-economic climate.

Because the cause so occupies and envelops those who have been bereaved by suicide, and will not go away, it would obviously be a great relief if the cause could be located and then neatly put away somewhere. Those bereaved by suicide particularly value the counselling they receive. It is essential that we highlight, during the time around the death, that their difficulties need immediate help.

One evening several years ago, a gentleman returned to me very distressed. He was sent back to the hospital because his family did not know what to do with him. He was inconsolable.

'This morning, I went round to my brother's house because

I had not seen him for a few days. He lived alone and had bouts of depression. He was a very private solitary sort of man but he had told me I was his best friend. That was hard for him to say.

We had a lot in common. We didn't have to say it but we both loved each other and had an understanding. I had recently gone through a divorce. He listened, and understood how bad things had been for me. The rest of the family commented on how we looked after each other. "You are the only one to get near him," they said.

Over the past week he had been a bit miserable. He sometimes went like that and sort of hibernated for a week, and I would go round and cheer him up if I could. I had a key to his house. I was the only one allowed to. He trusted me.

When I unlocked the door and walked into the hall I thought there was a funny smell. Then I saw him. It was grotesque, unbelievable, he was hanging from the bannister. He looked horrible. He was clearly dead and I wanted to run up to him and hold him and shout: No, Why? You'll be all right. Don't, please. The other part of me made me run, I ran out of the house and fell to the ground, unable to speak. I thought I was choking.

There were people standing over me looking down, and I thought: In a minute I will wake up from this horrible nightmare. An ambulance came and they laid me on a stretcher and carried me into it. It was all real: You are awake, I told myself, It is all real. I started to shake and then cry, and I could not stop.

When they took me home from the hospital my parents, brother and sisters said: "He has taken it very hard." Taken it hard, for God's sake, what do they expect? They said I should talk to you because I couldn't speak. Well, here I am talking away without stopping.

It was when they said "He has taken it hard." If I had spoken then they would not have known what hit them. Yes, I have taken it hard. He said he loved me and I was his only friend. He knew I had a key and would find him like that. How can anyone do that to someone?

I hate him. He was a liar to say I was his only friend. You don't do that to friends. I hate the swine and I hope he rots in hell. I will never recover from this, ever. How could you?

Yes, they were right to say I couldn't speak, because if I had they would have heard something they didn't like. How could I do that to my mother. Now I am bad, a wicked person, hating my poor sad brother. What a mess, what an absolute mess.'

He cried for a long time and I held him, and he returned several times to become reconciled to his beloved brother. This reconciliation, even after death, allowed him to begin to live again without him.

As you will appreciate from that one incident, there are many issues to work through, and their avoidance can prevent progress through the grief process. Opportunity must be given to deal with the immense and irrational guilt which is invariably a problem.

The behavior of the deceased prior to suicide has often caused severe relationship difficulties, so life prior to the death has been very stressful. So it is to be expected that this long period of stress, compounded by the suicide, must be one of the most traumatic events one could possibly have to cope with.

Whilst suicide is an intentional act performed by a person to end their own life, there are other types of self-destruction. Other sudden deaths may contain an element of self-destruction, and the bereaved may need further help. This may be apparent at the time of the death and, if it is, it will be an issue in the later stages of grieving.

Overeating, smoking, working too hard, hazardous sports or hobbies or reckless driving may result in untimely death. Relatives left in the immediate throes of the loss may well express anger:

'Why did he work so hard? He drove himself to this. The doctor told him to stop smoking but he wouldn't. He has only himself to blame.'

'He knew that racing would kill him one day. He almost expected it. What does that say about him and me?'

The feeling that relatives are left with problems, which in some way leaves them devalued by the deceased, is a painful issue to deal with. There was evidence that this difficulty was confronted at the time of death, and remained an area to be explored when we saw them later.

So, even if you are not working with definite suicide, the contribution of some people to their own death may be a counselling point.

Not only is death by suicide untimely, but there are cultural taboos and religious difficulties which can prevent or inhibit expressions of grief. The other ingredients of ambivalence, particularly associated with the pre-death stress, are a mixture of relief and sadness.

Most people bereaved by suicide feel abandoned to sort out this mess, and devalued by the deceased. In my opinion, suicide always and without doubt needs some counselling support. It would take a very competent, capable individual to handle the psychological difficulties alone.

VIEWING THE BODY

When relatives were seen later they talked of the definite value of contact with the deceased. Whilst some of this subject is covered previously, other points are worth noting.

Because relatives may not be present at the point of death, but only after death has been declared, viewing the body is especially valued. The chance to say 'I am sorry I was not with you,' and to affirm the death, was later described as providing comfort. It was interesting that the place they saw the deceased was commented upon later.

It is important to see the deceased where they died. This may be a resuscitation room or treatment room. Some saw the body again later, in the chapel next to the hospital mortuary, but said they were comforted by being able to see them where they had died. This somehow takes the bereaved closer to the event, and they have a strong need to feel part of it. There was not one negative response to viewing the body.

When Marjorie Ashdown and I did a phone-in on local radio about sudden death, most of the problems phoned about concerned the absence of a body. One lady rang to say her son was lost overboard at sea 20 years ago, and she still expected him to walk through the door. Wives of pilots missing in the war talked of their difficulty at not having a body to see and confirm death by.

There was a debate about bringing the bodies of the dead from the Falklands war back to Britain, which highlighted the value of the focus on the body. Raphael (1986) in her experiences with bereavement, and particularly disaster, pointed out that not being able to see the body contributes to the difficulties experienced by the bereaved later.

Whilst Cathcart (1988) says that relatives' reluctance to see the body should be respected, she goes on to say they should be encouraged to view and that photographs should be kept.

I am much happier with our current assertive response to this. Our previous response to the question of 'Should I see the body?' was a passive one:

> 'You can if you want to.'
> 'It is your decision.'

I have no hesitation now in saying:

> 'Yes, I think you should.'

We can make it a most natural thing to do:

> 'I am sure you would want to see him, even if it's only to say goodbye.'

Occasionally I hear of someone regretting seeing the deceased, but these regrets are unusual. There are more regrets and difficulties arising from not seeing the body, and later it is, of course, too late. The risk of regret is worth taking as a beneficial outcome is far more likely.

A study by Jones & Buttery (1981) of relatives of sudden death victims who spent time with the body in the Emergency Department, concluded that the viewing process was helpful. Most stated that the whole episode seemed like a fantasy or a bad dream, and that the viewing made it a reality. Reality, whilst painful, is more manageable than fantasy.

Several people in our study who did not see the body had difficulties with fantasies of how it looked. Fantasies can hold you and are less controllable, whilst reality is preferable and frees you from bizarre and distressing images.

People found it helpful that, if for example, someone was blue-looking after death, this was pointed out before they saw

the body. In cases of head and facial injures you would, perhaps, think it wiser to prevent someone from seeing the body.
This is not so, as long as people are told before going in to
view. If necessary the injuries can be covered, and it need not
prevent them holding the deceased's hand.

Viewing the body was a major issue in our feedback from
relatives. It affirmed for me that the time and effort spent with
relatives and the deceased are tremendously valuable in
providing some comfort at a most difficult period. There
seems little doubt that it helps to begin the process of grief,
and it was important to us as a team, in the Accident and
Emergency Department, to have that sort of positive feedback.

THE CONCLUDING TRANSACTION

Relatives told us how, after news of the death was given and
they had viewed the body, they had then to leave and go
home. We have noticed that there is, of course, a reluctance
to do this. How can you leave the person behind? It has been
clear to us for a long time that people may need help to leave,
and yet do not want to feel they are being rushed out. One
of the anxieties about offering people the opportunity to sit
with the body was that they would not want to leave. This
rarely happens, but if it does it should be openly discussed.

Part of the concluding process may be to sign for and take
away valuables such as rings or a watch, or signing for and
receiving clothing. Information on how to contact the coroner,
or obtain a death certificate bring the transaction to a more
practical level. People realise they have to go home and, on a
practical level, make arrangements for a funeral or to take up
life without the deceased.

People appear to need a clear indication that they can leave.
After being asked if there are any questions left unanswered
they actually do need permission to leave. No dissatisfaction
was expressed about this at follow up.

As a result of our study, we now offer people the facility of
returning, either soon or in the longer term, to discuss any
outstanding issues. This offer is often accepted. The card
given to them with the telephone number of the hospital and
the coroner also states the name of the nurse looking after

them, so that they can quickly identify and contact directly the key individual involved.

Careful records need to be kept, as some people may contact the hospital a year later. Whilst the nurse involved is likely to have retained a great deal of information, if he or she has left, good records are essential.

The relatives' evaluation of how we viewed their emotional response to the loss will be explored in more detail in the next chapter. Although in many ways it fits in to this review of the events that day, it also fits in with our difficulties with these responses.

Some of the insights into these responses, gained on retrospective evaluation, may help us to feel more comfortable about them. In the next chapter, we will therefore identify the responses that proved most difficult for us, but then describe how relatives later felt about this response of theirs. How they viewed our difficulty with them is important.

I want to repeat at this stage how grateful I am to those relatives who agreed to share their experiences of this painful and difficult time. It has been a great help for evaluating how we can care more effectively for people in this situation.

For us who work with the pain and distress, it has validated our efforts and commitment to it. We have also been reminded that we have much to learn about the process and immediate care, if we choose to listen.

I am often asked if the work is depressing. Hearing of some of the terrible and overwhelming difficulties of people, and how they overcome them, is far from depressing. It highlights the resourcefulness, courage, and lots of care and support that is available both from family and friends, or from professionals.

How we use the insights gained is examined in the next half of the book, which concentrates on the role of the carer.

REFERENCES

Bowlby J 1981 Sadness and depression. Attachment and loss, vol 3. Penguin, Harmondsworth
Cathcart F 1988 Seeing the body after death. British Medical Journal 297: 997–998
Cook B, Philips S G 1988 Loss and bereavement. Austin Cornish, London
Durkheim E 1951 Suicide. The Free Press, New York

Freud S 1917 Mourning and melancholia, standard edn, vol XIV. Hogarth, London

Henley S 1983 Bereavement by suicide. Bereavement care, vol 2, Cruse, London

Jones W H, Buttery M 1981 Sudden death — survivors' perceptions of their emergency department experience. Journal of Emergency Nursing 7: 1

Kübler-Ross E 1969 On death and dying. Macmillan, New York

Kübler-Ross E 1975 Death — the final stages of growth. Prentice Hall, New Jersey

Onions C T 1983 The shorter Oxford English dictionary. Oxford University Press, Oxford.

Parkes C M 1975 Bereavement: studies of grief in adult life, 2nd edn. Penguin, Harmondsworth

Raphael B 1986 When disaster strikes. Hutchinson, London

Wordon J W 1983 Grief counselling and grief therapy. Tavistock, London

4

What incapacitates the carer?

One of the benefits of our study was that it helped to identify some of the difficulties for the carer. Certain emotional responses from relatives of sudden death victims are more likely than others to leave the carer distressed or feeling ineffective. We were able to identify what these responses were when the immediate news of a sudden death was given.

On reflection, you may feel that despite our knowledge of these responses and insight into the process of grieving, we nevertheless have to make contact with the raw feelings. This will hurt or be painful irrespective of how much knowledge we have. That hurt, that encounter with grief on its impact, is very distressing and disruptive, and we have discussed the disorder that results.

Some insights into what can leave us feeling ineffective, or into what lies behind this response in the relative, can make the whole thing much more manageable for the carer. It will somehow lessen the feeling of chaos and disorder because we can identify the response either at the start of or during the process of grieving.

Whilst the primary focus of this chapter is to examine what incapacitates the carer, how the clients felt about their immediate response at a later date will be clarified. The emotional stance he takes on impact, the particular response that emerges, or how he defends himself at this time, can give some insight into the person and his struggles with the grief. Whilst responses are certainly not clarified as right or wrong, some will need more working with immediately and will be less well received by the person from whom they emerge. It will also be of interest that what makes carers uncomfortable may contain a more beneficial aspect for the client, whilst what carers find acceptable or easier to manage will create difficulty for the client. Crying was the only exception to this.

Another result that emerged from the study was that the client is aware of the carer's difficulties. What we the carers identified as making us uncomfortable or at a loss with the clients later identified and were extremely accurate about. This taught me that we should be more honest and use our difficulties together with the clients':

'The sister in Casualty who told me my husband was dead was very nice, but she could not cope with it. I had a feeling she would be glad when I left and went home. Several times she said, "You don't want to hang around here, you will be better off at home."

Later she said, "Your friends at home will look after you."

I could not take it in. He was a young man, 36 years of age, fit and well. Out jogging and he just dies. I did not want to rush off home. My head was in turmoil. It did not make any sense. I asked her several times if it was true and she became more and more fidgety and distressed. I had seen him dead but thought perhaps it was a nightmare. I wanted to see again if it was true but I knew I was becoming a nuisance.

I suppose it's just in one door, not saved, dead, out of the other door, get the relatives home, ready for the next one. I am not blaming her really but she should have given me more time. I thought afterwards that she probably had a husband the same age as mine. She just could not cope with it.'

This illustrates how this nurse's difficulty was apparent to the client. This lady was quite accurate in saying that the sister was in a hurry to get her home. When I interviewed the sister, within 24 hours of the death, she admitted to her difficulty with the lady and her haste to get her off home.

The other issue was that this nurse did have a husband the

same age as the client's husband, just as the client had pointed out. He too was an avid jogger, and the whole scenario confronted the sister with her own worst fears. If she had been able to recognise this, she would have compensated for it and given the lady more objective and effective care.

How we prepare staff to recognise these problems will be explored in the chapter on teaching and training for the work.

The nurses in our study identified in relatives nine emotional responses to the news of the sudden death. Obviously people experienced and displayed more than one feeling at the same time, although one may have been predominant. Some people experienced opposite ends of the spectrum of emotions, such as acceptance and then denial.

The survey results in Boxes 4.1 and 4.2 show the different responses seen in the key person at the time of the death, the number of people expressing them, and the degree of difficulty that nurses had in dealing with them.

Withdrawal
Denial
Anger
Isolation
Bargaining
Inappropriate responses
Guilt
Crying, sobbing, weeping
Acceptance

Box 4.1 Emotional responses to a sudden death — in descending order of difficulty for the nurses in the survey.

Withdrawal	30
Denial	28
Anger	27
Isolation	24
Bargaining	23
Inappropriate responses	13
Guilt	12
Crying, sobbing, weeping	11
Acceptance	3

Box 4.2 Emotional responses to 100 studied deaths. *Note:* many of the bereaved displayed more than one emotion.

You will see that withdrawal produced the most difficulty and acceptance, crying and sobbing produced the least.

We will look at each response separately to explore what we mean by it. How the significant relative perceived this response in retrospect will also be discussed. I have since discovered that talking over how people reacted emotionally on impact produces a useful way of exploring the grief.

WITHDRAWAL

This is where the client becomes inaccessible, mute, and appears to be refusing to listen. This response leaves the carer questioning her effectiveness. Since this result came out of the study I have checked this reponse in other disciplines, particularly those caring for the bereaved. In these workshop settings the effect of this response on the carer has become apparent:

'You wonder if you could have cared for them better.'
'It makes you question the communication skills you have for these situations.'
'You are just left looking at them, feeling helpless.'

If this is explored further with the carer, another difficulty that emerges is the silence. This can be particularly uncomfortable for nurses, whose ethos is about working, caring, or being busy. Nurses have great difficulty in seeing the value of just being there without putting it right. It is not like being able to put a bandage on and 'making it better'. The wound is deep and painful and the attempt at first aid appears to produce poor results.

Long periods of silence are perceived as sitting doing nothing. The carer searches around for something to do or say. Her efforts appear to fall on deaf ears. The silence is seen as being of little value though the client perceives it differently, as will be seen later.

The carer feels very vulnerable. This space or time may become a period of self-confrontation as she waits for a response from the client. Several nurses said they started to think what they would do if they were in the client's place.

Others described thinking for the first time in a long while about issues such as how can God allow this. Another common thought was how painful and unjust this death was, and how can anyone survive such an experience.

The withdrawal and the space it provides can therefore leave the carer confronting herself with some very difficult thoughts to wrestle with.

A common thought occurring to carers in this situation was that perhaps this person does not want me — the withdrawal was seen as rejection. They felt they obviously had very little to offer and this led them to wonder whether the client should be left alone. Is the withdrawal a way of saying 'leave me alone'.

As you can see, withdrawal leaves carers feeling they have little to offer and are ineffective. As if this were not enough, they themselves might begin confronting some difficult questions concerning the meaning of life. There was no hesitation in our group of nurses (and since in other disciplines) in saying that withdrawal was difficult to tolerate and understand.

The relatives' perception of withdrawal

'I remember it as if it was yesterday. When they said my son was dead I couldn't speak or move. It struck me down somehow, except I was just sitting there. I remember the nurse. She looked helpless and I thought, "She wants me to do something but what can I do?"

I do not remember how long it lasted but his whole life went before me. Some of it was lovely and made me smile. She (the nurse) looked puzzled as if I was going mad. She got hold of my hand but I was locked into some sort of memory — she's talking about my boy, my son, the first child I gave birth to. I watched him grow, take his first steps. I laughed when he got his words all mixed up.

Dead. What can she mean? This is the boy who was so scared the first day he went to school, but so brave. He could run, run like a hare. How proud he was of his medals. He cannot be dead.

She does not know him. This is my son you are talking about. He was not that clever at school but when he left he was doing all right. That day he brought home his first girl friend. He was shy and embarrassed but tried to be the big, macho man. He was a man, but he cried 6 months later when she left him.

This is my son they are talking about. Dead. "Yes," she said, "the worst has happened. He has died."'

Mrs Brown described her withdrawal. It actually lasted for 20 minutes as noted on the initial evaluation of her care. This is a long time to sit in silence whilst someone rocks and smiles to herself occasionally.

When we saw Mrs Brown later she did not know about the time lapse. She described how, on impact, she retraced her life with her son, how she tried to make sense of it and how this retracing helped. It brought her back to the present, to the pain and awful impact. She needed this retracing to help her understand what was happening.

Mrs Brown remembered the nurse's discomfort with her withdrawal. She was not critical of her because of this, and said, 'I'm so glad she was there with me.' This confirms the value of being able to stay with the pain and distress. That is no easy task. It takes some doing particularly for those who are new to caring for people in this way. When the nurse left the room and she was alone, Mrs Brown was scared. She hoped she would return soon.

There is tremendous value, therefore, in being able to stay with withdrawal, and our presence is a comfort and strength. We must not make the assumption that no response means rejection and leave the client alone. Check this out first. Unless they can clearly verbalise that they want to be alone, stay with them.

The retracing that takes place silently in so many people is important. It helps them to understand the death in the context of the whole of their loved one's life. It is the beginning of exploring its meaning, and confronting its pain and disorder. When the client eventually re-emerges from the withdrawal, he or she may begin to tell you about their retracing of steps in the deceased's life. Again this is an important step in the process of grieving.

To know the value of being there, without this being immediately validated, is important to the carer. This knowledge makes the transaction more manageable.

DENIAL

Denial of the fact or feelings of the death is denial of its reality. In withdrawal, the reality is accepted and work can begin on this. Denial can be clearly expressed as the death not being wanted or acceptable:

> 'Don't you dare say he is dead.'
> 'Go away. That cannot be true. I will just go home and forget this.'

Sometimes the fact may be received but the feelings of denial that emerge may surprise the client:

> 'How can I be feeling this?' is a common question. Others comment on the experience being new:
> 'I have never felt anything like this before. It cannot be true.'
> 'These feelings are not mine.'
> 'This is not a part of my life.'
> 'You must have the wrong person, this is not part of my life scheme or plan. Go away and find the right person.'

The awful imposition of this death onto the person, and the way it interferes with future plans or schemes, is very marked here.

If the denial is quickly dissipated it is a relief for the carer but means the enormity and impact have been received. If the denial persists, the carer will question her ability to communicate effectively, is also frustrated by this ineffectiveness and may become more forceful or directive. The carer is left in the invidious position of having to reiterate or reinforce some painful and distressing information.

If someone leaves the scene or hospital in a rigid state of denial we rightly feel anxious about them. This rarely happens, and usually we establish death's awful reality quickly.

Most nurses who give news of sudden death expect denial. They also expect to deal with this and help people to accept death's reality. If denial persists for 5 minutes or more nurses become uncomfortable. The person receiving the painful information will ask you to say it is not true. It is difficult and uncomfortable for the bearer of the news to have to confirm the pain which is clearly distressing.

There is little wonder then, that denial in relatives rates high as a cause of distress in the carer, when all the carer can do is reinforce the relatives' distress. Nurses see themselves in this act of confirmation as piling on the agony. One nurse described it as being like 'kicking someone when they are down'.

Many of the relatives, evaluated in the immediate situation as displaying marked denial that persisted and was difficult to work with, showed evidence of this in the later visit. Remember, some were seen at 6 months and others at 10 months. There was evidence that this initial denial and difficulty was still a persistent theme later. One nurse said:

'I remember Mrs X just would not accept the death of the baby. Her husband and father-in-law colluded with this. When I suggested that she should see and hold the baby they were angry. They were really saying she cannot cope with this, as you can see by the way she is denying it, and still you suggest that.

It was as though I was just adding to her distress, but I felt it was right. She sat and held him, and rocked backwards and forwards, talking to him and then said, "Let's just go home and forget all this. I just want to take my baby home."

I said, "It can't ever be the same, he is dead," and she cried and said, "I know, I just wanted to bury him in the garden so he is near me."

Her husband said, "Look what you have done."' '

The relatives' perception of denial

When Mrs X was seen later she had left the denial and had begun to grieve about her baby's death. A definite indication from her was that the nurse had helped her a lot. She perceived the immediate struggle with denial as madness.

The struggle for the carer is in helping the client to find acceptable something that is more than just difficult information. It is helping them to see clearly something that penetrates into their very being. It has to make us question what we are doing.

Comment on both aspects of denial

Many people remembered the denial and how they struggled with it, but also how death's awful reality was quickly a part of their existence. Those who struggled with its reality were also aware of this struggle persisting, and many made this connection themselves.

It is useful in the longer term counselling relationship to explore this immediate difficulty and how it was dealt with at the time or not dealt with. Useful parallels can be drawn as to how they are working with it now.

ANGER

However shortlived the experience, anger can be frightening; it can push people away from each other leaving each alone and vulnerable. People who are angry lose intellectual clarity and reasoning powers, and are consumed by this powerful emotion.

Anger in grief gives glimpses of its nature at both ends of the spectrum. In its mild form people are irritated and, at the other end of the continuum, in a rage. Irritation is often due to some aspect of loss on the periphery away from the main focus (Fig. 4.1), and we may feel this response is inappropriate:

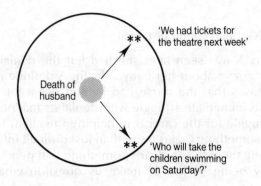

Figure 4.1 Major focus and flight to periphery.

This lady sidestepped the major focus of her crisis — her husband's death — to some irritating aspects of her loss somewhere on the periphery. When she returned to the major focus of her crisis she experienced rage.

Many people label the anger as anxiety or fear, because this seems much more acceptable to them and others, including the carer. The anger is seen as destructive and wicked or sinful. For some reason anger is rejected or mistrusted, and not seen as the warning device that it is. Anger can be expressed verbally and its catharsis produces solutions.

Rage is much more a physical expression and its release is usually damaging. In grief, rage adds to the torment and is a terrifying experience for the carer. For a long time we had a hole in the wall of our relatives' room. This was the result of a father's anger at the death of his son in a road traffic accident and someone mentioning that the driver had been going too fast.

Whilst this kind of anger produces fear and panic, it does not produce the most difficulty as anger directed towards the carer is fairly well accepted, though not easy. It may be an indication of our personality types that we expect to suffer a little in this role. The anger that makes us most distressed or uncomfortable is anger directed towards the deceased:

On being told of the death of his son in a motor cycle accident, Mr B said:
'He always was an idiot and now he's gone and got himself killed. You spend all your time working for them, to give them everything, and they do this to you. I will never forgive him for this, never. I hate him.'
When the nurse suggested he did not really mean this and he would see things differently later, he told her to shut up.
'What do you know about it, anyway?' he responded angrily. 'Mind your own business.'
The nurse was very distressed and later described a strong need to defend this person who was unable to defend himself. She also thought his father would regret saying these things, and attempted to put him right.

To return to the type of people carers are, again we often take responsibility for how people feel, and in defending the deceased we feel pushed into verbally defending someone who is unable to defend himself. This highlights some issues that may need clarifying and exploring before we undertake bereavement counselling. It begs the question about who is responsible for whom, and how the work can be a heavy burden.

Anger directed at the health care system, the doctor or the nurse, was much more acceptable than anger at the deceased. In my group of nurses, it was interesting how many were prepared for anger being directed at them but were surprised and distressed at its being directed at the deceased. To many of them this seemed inappropriate.

If relatives directed anger towards themselves, carers were able to work with this and usually offer some reassurance, though less easily if the deceased had committed suicide.

The relatives' perception of their anger

Where anger had been a clear response in the immediate situation, it remained a difficulty. The focus of the anger may have changed during the 6 or 10 months' interval, but it remained a difficulty to work with. If the anger had been directed at the deceased, the relative apologised for this and was embarrassed. One lady who was angry with her husband for working too hard and killing himself as a result of stress, had changed the focus of the anger when seen later:

'I blame his bosses for letting him work like he did. It was only to line their pockets. They reaped all the benefit. Only I was the loser, and him of course. They robbed me of all we had planned for his retirement. That was to be ours and they took it all. I despise the management. I suppose the hate I feel for them is burning me up inside. Just talking about it now could drive me to murder.

If my family knew I was talking like this they would disown me. They say he was a wonderful husband and I should just be thankful for this. Sometimes I think if I had a gun I would have committed murder. I suppose you think I am awful.'

Most people are ashamed of this anger and really value the opportunity of discussing it.

Comment on both perceptions of anger

In a counselling relationship, this anger can usually be shared and seen as an expression of the despair of the loss. Sudden death produces a fight to understand and control the grief of the loss and this produces anger. We must be careful not to impose our own feelings about what is appropriate on others, as we remember our own family messages about anger and how and where it should be expressed.

Anger was in the top three emotional responses producing difficulties for the carer. Many carers, including my nurse group and others from workshops, have expressed fear of being hurt physically when working with sudden death. Few were prepared for this being a possibility.

ISOLATION

Feelings of isolation as expressed by the relatives remind us of our own vulnerability should we be bereaved and left alone. Obviously this is frightening for the carer but nurses did not find this to be the major difficulty with the bereaved person's sudden sense of isolation. The nurses were most uncomfortable for and with the other people (friends or relatives) surrounding the key person.

When the key person was given the news of the sudden death or this was confirmed, he or she experienced a sudden sense of isolation or being alone. This was in spite of being surrounded by significant and caring people. For example, a common response to the loss of a spouse was:

> 'I am all alone now.'
> 'I have nobody.'

If this was followed by another comment about being powerless and helpless, such as:

> 'All my strength has gone.' or
> 'I have nothing left, nothing to go on for.'

friends and relatives quickly want to assure them of their love and support:

> 'We will be with you .'

'You have all your family and friends.'

'You will not be alone.'

Despite these assurances the bereaved person continues to express a total loss, and feelings of being totally alone and isolated. The distress for the carer appears to stem from the inability of those closest to comfort the bereaved, and from witnessing their distress about this. The carer also feels ineffective as she reminds the bereaved of what he has left, because this appears to give little comfort.

The carer is simply left to sit and look upon a person's overwhelming sense of isolation, where everyone around him, despite strong reassurances of their presence, appear to have little to offer.

In Kübler-Ross's book, *To Live Until We Say Goodbye (1978)*, she describes this sense of isolation, along with denial, as a mechanism to defend until resources can be mobilised. She describes it as a buffer allowing the client to pull himself together and mobilise alternative defences.

In my longer-term counselling, clients have described how, although it distresses friends and relatives, the bereaved needs people to know that no other person has on offer what the deceased had to give them. The powerful and central message at this time is that no-one can replace this person or stand in for them, so do not try.

When those closest to the bereaved state plainly that they cannot give or have on offer what the deceased did, this becomes less of an issue.

The relatives' perception of feeling isolated

A young lady, whose husband died suddenly at the age of 39 from a heart attack, described how she suddenly felt isolated. She also knew when seen later, that her expression of this had distressed those around her.

'When they said he was dead it was the strangest experience. It was just like being in a big open space, a bit like a desert. It even felt dry and desolate. All these people were around me, my mother and father and brother, and they were

all saying we will take care of you. I remember saying, "You cannot, nothing will help me with this."

I was totally alone. There was nothing I or anyone could do. All their words were useless, they were just words. What could they do? I had lost everything. There was nothing left. The more they tried to reassure me the worse it became. I know I just looked, as much as to say "You have nothing for me."

Nothing can comfort or console you when you have lost everything.'

It is not at all unusual for the client to perceive the loss as total. Whatever they have acquired is of no consolation. Even more painful for those close to them is that they are not seen as a resource. The message they receive is that there is nothing they can offer to help with this. It is difficult for them to be left feeling as helpless as this, and difficult for the carer to witness this predicament.

Comment on these perceptions of isolation

We are again reminded, when confronted with this most distressing emotional response, of our inability to put it right. The particular difficulty for doctors and nurses is that in distressing conditions there is often something they can do to offer a crumb of comfort. But here you cannot get near the person, they feel totally alone and you are not seen as a resource.

One of the lessons we have to learn in the caring professions is that we do not always have some prescription to put things right, and that there are some intensely distressing situations where we can only stay and observe. Eventually, when they are ready, people will begin to emerge from this powerful sense of isolation and will need some resources. We have somehow to wait on the outside of the pain and be ready to step forward to help and support.

Some people emerge from the feeling of isolation very quickly — that is, within 10 or 15 minutes of impact of death — only to return to this state later. Some describe this as returning to how they felt at the time. It may be that the impact of the enormity of the loss has to be confronted again before some people can begin to explore other resources. As our group of carers was reminded, it is distressing to witness and leaves us feeling helpless.

BARGAINING

Bargaining in sudden death is where the client attempts to postpone the death by formulating an agreement. He may think that if he alters his behaviour he will prevent the death or be granted an 'extension'. I have witnessed this response most often when the death of a child or young person is involved.

When death is imminent, or news of the death is about to be given and they are aware of what you are about to say, the bargaining begins. This, in my experience, is usually about reconciliation with someone they are estranged from, particularly where parents are separated or divorced. There may be remorse for bad behaviour or separation from God. The bargaining may be directed to a specific person or to anyone in the room; some people look heavenward as if appealing to God, whilst others address God by name:

'If you put this right God, I will not let you down again.'
'I will return to the church. I'm sorry, please help me.'

Husbands or wives, or other family members, may appeal to each other:

'From now on we must try to stop arguing and care for our family better. We have failed them. I promise if this can be put right we will all care for each other better.'

Some doctors and nurses are distressed that people will bargain with them for a life:

'I will give you all my money, all I have, if you will save him.'
'No expense must be spared, bring the best people you have. I will find the money somehow. I will sell all I have.'

Despite assurances that the best possible expertise will not save this life, or that the child is already dead, the bargaining may persist. This type of bargaining leaves the carer feeling very uncomfortable, and some are clearly distressed with the idea that money could be an issue in the saving of a life.

Other workers, particularly if they are parents themselves, are distressed at witnessing parents exhorting each other to promise to be good, and having the idea that their bad behaviour has brought this tragedy upon them. In one discussion group a nurse stated that it reminds you of the frailty and vulnerability of intimate relationships. She did not want any suggestion that the stability of these relationships had an effect on life or death outcomes.

The relatives' perception of bargaining

I have counselled several parents who clearly remember bargaining, and I suspect there are many more bargains secretly made with God. Some people admit to this, but with hindsight feel foolish about it. It is important that with hindsight and after counselling, they usually have a greater sense of our inability to control matters of life and death.

If the counselling has been useful, there will have been a shift from how we control or influence these issues, to what we gain from life each day. Many of the parents I know who have bargained describe it as a desperate attempt to regain control of the situation. They describe a sudden chaos being imposed upon them, and a need to find a solution to restore order. Alongside this is a desperate need for explanations, for answers to why this is happening.

This need produces a possible explanation — they themselves must have erred from the straight and narrow and their bad behaviour, sin or wickedness has caused this to happen. They then quickly bargain to put this right. Many hours are spent with these people, particularly parents, exploring the meaning of the death and whether it is the outcome of some bad behaviour or sin.

Some parents actually apologise because they have been selfish in that they were too happy with their children. Others reprimand themselves for never having given a thought to the fact that their child may die, and why should it only happen to others and not theirs. Their search through these issues may be the outcome of their initial bargaining.

Comment on these responses to bargaining

It would appear that most carers, although experiencing some distress in these situations, are able to respond to them. They can provide reassurance that everything is being done or has been done to save the life, and are able to ask people not to blame themselves and to remind them it was an accident or something they could not foresee. Most carers will want to give these assurances quickly, and will therefore be able to offer a response and not be left feeling helpless as in some of the previous responses.

When parents are begging forgiveness of each other, with promises to be better in future, this is more distressing. Not only is there an exchange of intimacies that you feel you are intruding upon, but it is difficult to break into and put right. This aspect of bargaining has been the most distressing for the carer.

INAPPROPRIATE RESPONSE

This is where the emotional response to the news of death appears inappropriate for the situation, as perceived either by the carer or the person receiving the bad news. Many individuals are immediately concerned at their lack of response and may state, alarmed:

'Why am I not feeling anything?'
'Should I be going mad now, or breaking down or something?'

In our study, such responses were recorded as inappropriate in the perception of the carer. Most of the situations where this was recorded were in the responses of an adolescent; something was blurted out which the speaker usually regretted immediately and apologised for, or which produced an angry response from another family member.

John was 15 years old and sat waiting with his father for news of his brother. Simon was 18, and he had only had the motor bike for a month. Now he was lying in the hospital, badly injured. Simon had worked hard to save up for that bike, John thought.

'Will the bike be OK?' John asked his father, when they were both told that Simon might die from his injuries.

'Don't be stupid, John,' his father replied angrily.

Simon wouldn't think it was stupid, John thought, wondering what to say next and not knowing whether to laugh or cry at his father's anger. He often laughed at it lately. He wanted to cry but did not know what to do with his Dad. He had never seen him like this before. He wondered if he should hold his hand, but then thought the nurse might think he was soft.

The doctor came in looking very serious, and began to talk, and his words did not come out properly. How awful, thought John, having a stutter and having to talk to people like this. He half smiled to himself and then saw everyone looking at him disapprovingly.

'I am very sorry, but Simon has just died,' the doctor said to John's father.

John did not know what to do. He felt he had not been told, although he was there. He was desperate to help. My Dad is in such pain, and here am I sitting doing nothing. Please God, tell me what to do, he thought. Give me Simon back. Put it right. After what seemed like an eternity in time, with John looking round the room for something to concentrate on, he said:

'I will have a room of my own now.'

With all eyes accusingly on him, he smiled weakly and wished the floor would open and swallow him up.

The relatives' perception of this response

People who experienced the wrong thoughts or words emerging describe later how uncomfortable, embarrassed and distressed they felt about this. They were often young adolescents struggling to understand how to cope with new and difficult feelings. These feelings were powerful and overwhelmed them, and produced a new and unknown fear.

They also describe an intense pressure to help to put things right. They describe having to respond to reactions in parents that they have never seen or experienced before. More painfully, for many bizarre reasons, many adolescents wonder if they are ultimately responsible. John from the last case study wondered whether it was because 3 days previously, in a discussion with his friend, he had said that God did not exist. Another explanation, given to me by a 14-year-old girl whose older sister had died, was that she had not been doing her homework and had been told that no good would come of it.

This tremendous pressure to help and the desperate search for something to take away some of the pain results in remarks which are perceived as inept, to say the least, or stupid or even wicked.

The carer's role with this response

Our role is primarily to set a good model in our response to the remark, by not being judgemental. We can so easily diffuse some of the anger and difficulty by saying how hard it is to find ways to respond to death. We can say how we are sure they must be at a complete loss as to what to do or say next, and that it is the worst thing in the world for people to find right or proper responses to.

We need to say this. For young people, we need to be seen to be caring, and accepting of their response and difficulty. Adolescents find the situation most difficult — they are neither child nor adult; people do not know what to do with them and they do not know what to do with themselves.

Include them in the breaking of the bad news, in any discussion following it, and in viewing of the body. It is a painful and often lonely time for many young people.

We have already discussed the problem of anger. It would be very easy, and does often happen, that at the onset of grief everyone's anger is directed at an easy target — a scapegoat. The response that is labelled as inappropriate may act as the trigger for allowing the mechanism of 'scapegoating' to occur.

John could easily have been the target of everyone's anger. He needed help to cope with and understand his feelings and ambivalence. So does his family.

ACCEPTANCE

Acceptance is the term used by most people in grief work to describe the final stages of grieving. This is when the client has had sufficient time and has worked through the previous stages. Acceptance describes when most of the emotional pain has gone and the struggle with the loss is over.

It is difficult and a surprise to some carers that, on hearing the news of a sudden death, some people appear to accept and not struggle with this information. They are not in a state of denial, and their perception is not altered or impaired; they simply receive and accept the loss.

It may be that some previous, overwhelming loss has prepared them for this one. The experience may not be new and they therefore have a previous impact programmed into their experience; this can make this impact less powerful.

I have heard of people who, on being given news of a sudden death, talk of how they have discussed this very possibility with the deceased and have made contingency plans for it. There will therefore be people who know by experience that sudden death is a possibility in all our lives. Not only will they not have denied or avoided this, but will have had open discussion of its possibility with loved ones.

Others will have validated their love for each other prior to the event, along with the knowledge of death being a possibility, and will therefore have no unfinished business. By unfinished business, I mean that they feel there is nothing left unsaid or undone. Again people might find this difficult to believe, but some people do use opportunities to the full, and happily feel, even in this situation, a sense of having completed something.

You will remember from looking at crisis theory that one of the difficulties about a crisis may be that it is a new experience. Although the death may be sudden, past experience with a previous death may leave a person with a way of making it manageable so that it may not be so chaotic or disordered.

Carers' perception of acceptance

Because we usually see sudden death resulting in disorder, we may have difficulty with or feel uncomfortable with acceptance of the death on impact. Our experience of acceptance is that it is the final stage of grief, and because of this, most carers involved in the impact of the sudden death check out more than once that the client is not in a state of denial.

Perhaps this is right. There will be many carers who will remain uncomfortable because someone has been able to receive and usefully work with the impact of sudden death. We must remember that this is our problem.

GUILT

Remorse is what we are left with quite frequently after a sudden death. The feeling that we are in some way to blame for the death is very common. The most frequent expression of this is guilt at failing to act or respond usefully or effectively:

> 'I was too slow in calling the ambulance.'
> 'I should have made him see a doctor.'
> 'I didn't want to travel on the route on which he was killed.'
> 'I should have made him wait to drive. He was too tired'.

It may be that because the person is not there to take responsibility for himself, we have to take it for him. For some, it is disrespectful or culturally difficult to make negative remarks about dead people. This will not only produce problems in the immediate situation, but also in the later stages of grieving.

The death is often felt to be a punishment. The client is left with a feeling that he has behaved in a way that is inconsistent with his internal value system or conscience. Some will state that they have sinned against God and that this is the outcome. A voice inside them states that their behaviour needs correcting and that this death is the sign that confronts them with that. The sudden death, as the outcome or punishment, is the ultimate message or reminder of having done something wrong by commission or omission.

Guilt is not necessarily inappropriate, and carers describe this as being even more difficult. When a drunken driver kills a spouse or a friend, it is appropriate that they should feel bad about it. If a drunken driver kills himself, people feel guilty about being angry with him for being so stupid. It is very easy to feel guilty.

Many situations evoke feelings of guilt and present a challenge to work with, e.g. ill health, sexual activity, surviving an accident when others have died. Helping the client to learn to forgive himself or others, and move forward, is a challenge.

Whilst some guilt is appropriate, some is excessive for the situation, and unhealthy. Most carers will be aware that, on impact, it is not always apparent that we have done anything to help this. It should not prevent us from trying, as people will later use what was offered in their struggle with the guilt.

The difficulties of being the survivor of a sudden death, particularly an accident, may result in feelings of shame:

'I could have saved him.'
'It should have been me that died.'

If someone is found out and exposed, or if, in the review of the events, a person feels to blame, he is left with shame. I heard a disaster worker say, in working with survivors, that she had never encountered so much shame. Shame is about exposure to self and others, and about being looked at or having fingers pointed at you. Blame and its resulting shame may stem from being found out or the threat of being found out. Shame reflects the character of the person, and has consequences.

The other problem about guilt, in the immediate or long term, is that guilt may be the result of parental programming. Parental messages of 'should' and 'ought' act as a conscience, and you may be left believing that when anything goes wrong you are to blame.

What could be more wrong than a sudden death? In the immediate situation, the difficulty for carers is that they wonder where to begin with this powerful programming.

In the immediate situation of sudden deaths, nurses perceived that guilt became an issue in the majority of cases. It was certainly an issue for most clients in the long term. A question worth asking was: is that why they responded to our request for help in our study? Did it offer some way of making amends, or offer some help in the search to minimise the guilt?

Client's perception of guilt

Some clients had reason to feel guilty by reason of commission or omission. They will say they have to live with and work through this. Others describe being overwhelmed with guilt, and later with help from relatives and friends who said they were being excessively punitive and looking for an answer as to why it happened.

The search to understand the reason for the death quickly leads on to other issues related to guilt, to issues of how much control we have over our lives, and whether this is governed by good and evil.

For some, issues of good and evil are perfectly clear. If somebody's sudden death is the result of a crime it may be seen clearly as being due to evil, sin and wickedness. For others, the search for an answer gives them a need to place the sudden death in some clear category.

It is very difficult for people to be able to say:

'It was an accident, he was in the wrong place at the wrong time, we could not foresee this.'

We seem to have a need to feel that we control our destiny and have complete authority over what happens to us. The fact that we do not have this power can make us feel uneasy, uncomfortable or out of control.

The difficulty with guilt for the carer

One of the real difficulties in dealing with the client's guilt is the very private nature of it. Whilst they may reveal some of it, there is often a discomfort at having done so, and a reluctance to proceed further. We are naturally uncomfortable with this, as further questioning may make us and the client aware of guilt's oppressive nature and its shame.

If the guilt response is excessive, we may attempt to reduce its impact, but if the guilt appears wholly appropriate in our perception of the event, we may be reluctant to try to take it from the client or lessen its impact.

A common response from the carer (nurses in our study) about guilt on impact was the enormity of the problem. Many felt, quite rightly, that there were so many other immediate tasks that we could have some influence on and work effectively with, that guilt would remain a longstanding issue for the client to work with.

Despite this, we should address sensitively the issues linked with guilt, and not avoid them. I would suggest the feeling was wholly appropriate, by saying something to the effect of:

'That will be something you will need to think about, and perhaps talk to someone about.'

We should not, in a perfunctory sort of way, dismiss as wholly inappropriate, guilt issues that appear to be excessive for the situation. They are valid and a difficulty for the client, and the client must not be made to feel stupid about them. Failure to work with the guilt may prevent someone working through the grief process:

'You read so much these days about fats and cholesterols and how we should avoid them. I had read it all, and just ignored it. My husband was only young really. Well, 41 years is not old. He played football and was doing so when he died. He smoked and liked his beer, and he loved that fatty bit on the joint of meat. We used to kid him on about it, and say it will be the death of you yet, but never once believing it would.

The death certificate said something about fat in his arteries. I know it's stupid but I never did anything to prevent that. We just pay lip service to so much, but we do nothing about it. The morning he died I gave him a big, fatty bacon sandwich. He loved them.

The thought of it now makes me sick. Since reading that death certificate I have not bought any bacon. I avoid it like the plague in the supermarket. When the lads asked why we didn't have any, I went crackers and started shouting at them. They couldn't understand it.

That sandwich tipped the balance. It took him over the edge. It killed him in the end, and I gave him it.'

Guilt is an issue where we can have some positive influence over how it is worked with, from the impact of the sudden death through the grieving process.

There will be other situations where issues of blame and guilt, and who carries it, will prevent the grief process taking place. After these issues have been publicly discussed at inquests, there can be further progress in the grieving or an even firmer stance on blame and guilt.

Legal wrangling over compensation, and putting a monetary value on someone's life and death, can further complicate matters.

CRYING, SOBBING AND WEEPING

Catharsis, or the release of strong feelings, has long been considered an important component of the therapeutic process. Freud (1910) discovered that no lasting benefit was produced by an outpouring of feelings, but that the release reduced anxiety and depression.

Freud also observed that weeping motivated the client to remain in therapy. In my longer-term counselling of bereaved clients, I find they often feel they have achieved something if there is an overt outpouring of grief in the session.

It is not always clear what constitutes an emotional arousal. A short burst of crying, quickly controlled, may signify intense arousal in a shy, inhibited individual.

Crying, sobbing and weeping will produce very different responses from observers, depending on the culture and sex of the person expressing the feeling. In a Western culture most people will be more comfortable with this response in a woman. People continue to be embarrassed when men cry, and in particular men themselves if the others present are women. Some Asian groups of men will cry openly and comfortably together without women being present.

Despite the sexual and cultural differences, a common response to sudden death is crying, sobbing and weeping, and most people, including the person crying, have a sense of its appropriateness.

This sadness or grief, when expressed as crying or sobbing, is often felt to be a good thing, and people wait for it to happen. It is perceived as a release of pain and distress. Most of the anxiety about it is the question of when it will stop. Many express a fear of its being unending, and draining away energy. When it happens you could say the person is suffering, and yet it is greatly valued by both lay and professional people.

Control is a word often used in relation to expression of sorrow. Losing control of one's feelings, or the inability to keep them internalised, verges on madness for some people. Loss of emotional control can easily be equated with insanity.

The relatives' perception of crying

Most people, when seen later, felt they had no difficulty with this response. Alongside this emotional response they felt it was easier for people to care for and comfort them. Of all the emotional responses to sudden death, this was seen in a positive light. More people speak of the value of this than of any other response discussed. Crying, sobbing and weeping facilitated physical contact more than any other response.

The carer's view of crying

This response produced the least difficulty for the nurses in my study. It appealed to their need to feel useful, and gave them something to do in physically comforting weeping people. The other aspect of crying that made it feel more comfortable and manageable was that it was understandable. It was easily understood as a response to sudden death, and felt to be wholly appropriate.

A study by Brewis (1989) of police officers, and how they react to dealing with sudden death, showed the opposite response. Police officers were less able to cope with crying, sobbing and weeping, and found withdrawal more comfortable to tolerate.

This opposite effect on them compared to nurses was felt to be due to role and conditioning. Police officers are taught to apply the law and not allow emotional considerations to impair their judgement. This emotional distancing from the client takes place many times in their daily work. So withdrawal, and the distancing this produces, is tolerated more easily than crying which evokes a nurturing response that they are less comfortable with than the nurses.

This difference in how the person in the carer's role reacts will, of course, have implications in differing training needs.

Brewis' study, which concerns informing relatives about a sudden death, also highlighted that policemen experienced greater stress on receiving the call to visit a house than there was on breaking the bad news.

The only difficulty with crying, described by two or three young female nurses, was at witnessing men cry. They went on to say that it confronted them with the fact that their own fathers were vulnerable and could cry. They did not want to be reminded of this.

It must be re-stated that people do not always want physical contact or to be comforted. We must be prepared to be rejected.

In this chapter we have looked at emotional responses in relatives on impact of sudden death. We have not only identified what the carer has difficulty in responding to at this time, but also what problems, with hindsight, the client experienced in his own responses. In gaining some insight into what clients experienced with these emotional responses, and how they perceived the carer's response, we begin to demystify some of the skills and responses.

Knowing the emotional responses at the time of sudden death, and how these are perceived by all involved, can only increase our insight and effectiveness.

This move into increasing our knowledge of sudden death, and how to confront the emotional responses, takes us on to teaching and training for the work.

REFERENCES

Brewis T 1989 Stress and reactions of police officers when warning relatives of a sudden or unexpected death. Unpublished study for West Yorkshire Police for HND

Freud S 1910 Two short accounts of psycho-analysis. Reprinted 1966 Penguin, Harmondsworth

Kübler-Ross E 1978 To live until we say goodbye. Prentice-Hall, NJ

5

Teaching and training for the work

Clients' attitudes and responses to sudden death are diverse in nature, and although different from our own or from what we may have witnessed, they are equally valid. There is no right or wrong response to sudden death, and this will be the subject of many discussions on training sessions.

In training for and exploring responses of clients and ourselves, we are not talking about right or wrong responses, but about the nature of these responses. We are not even saying they can be described as aberrations or clinical signs of 'illness' but as human responses to an overwhelming difficulty.

The teaching and training are to help us to help them effectively. That may mean doing nothing, or nothing more than helping them to explore resources.

Some part of these difficult encounters, and how much power or control the carer can have in each situation, can be explored before the event. This will help us as carers to remain personally and professionally effective, when the very nature of the work can have the opposite effect and leave us feeling burnt out.

One of the aims of our teaching sessions will be to help the carers remain potent by re-arming themselves with insights and responses to the difficulties. It may be important, therefore, to give carers permission to have time out at the start of the session, to look at their own needs as well as those of the clients. It is often difficult for carers to do this, as it feels a little like self-indulgence.

Time out to explore the issues helps the carer to return to a position of strength. The need for this does not invalidate our other need to focus on and identify vulnerability.

During recent years of looking at the needs of the client and the carer, I have also been involved in training. This chapter examines some of the stated needs of people working with sudden death. It examines issues to be formally taught, particularly those in the first chapter, and describes games and exercises that focus on particular issues of communication and skill.

Whilst the success of some of these depends on particular groups and mixtures of disciplines or hierarchies, in general they provide a more informal and relaxed way of teaching a difficult subject. They are not set out in any particular order, but offered to be used in teaching and training sessions as appropriate.

It is worth stating that the very presence of the carers at a training session is a sign of their commitment to working with very difficult situations. Many will have lots of experience in this, and their presence is another chance for them to re-evaluate what they know, and to share it. It is often difficult in the work setting to look objectively at what we do and the knowledge we have acquired. The training session is to help us do just that.

POSITIVE AND NEGATIVE EXERCISE

To follow this thought through, ask them to produce a list of all that they bring into these situations that is positive, and then a list of what they feel is negative. When they have done this, and you have listed them on a board at the front of the room, ask them how it is that some things can be on both lists. An example of this may be:

Persistent encounters with death.

The mix of the workshop or study day between formal exposition of theories and less structured discussion also provides a useful balance. Totally open, unstructured days leave some learners so open and vulnerable that the experience becomes negative. A good mix will offer some safety, and perhaps the structure is something people will be comfortable with since school days.

BRAINSTORM

Issues linked with the need for structure to work with may be reflected in an early brainstorming exercise. Asking people quickly to identify their needs or what will help to equip them for the work can also highlight their expectations of themselves or of the day's training.

Below are some of the needs which are quickly identified at the start of these training days:

```
Interpersonal skills
Help with words to communicate
   sensitively
Help with feelings and attitudes
   of the bereaved
Insights into responses
Structured ways of working
Response to difficult behaviour
   such as anger or high activity
To be able to handle the stress
```

Box 5.1 Brainstorming — examples of needs commonly expressed.

Some of these key issues may need several sessions, and highlight deficiencies within the organisation. If, for example, the workshop is on the stresses of working with sudden death, use the brainstorm for another exercise.

Ask the group to identify from the list what may highlight organisational difficulties. This can be explored further by asking them to discuss, in small groups, what we as carers must take some personal responsibility for. It will be interesting to see how each group's spokesperson can offer such different ideas on this.

Give another group unlimited resources of people and money to take away into their group. Ask them to use this to set up good support structures for helping carers remain effective in the work of caring for the suddenly bereaved.

Give another group very limited resources. As these resources may not go far, instruct the group to use them effectively. Ask them to prioritise, with the greatest needs identified first. Compare the outcomes of both groups.

EXPLORING ISSUES INVOLVED IN COPING

In very simple terms, coping is about our response to change. Lazarus (1966), in his studies of coping behaviour, describes two aspects of coping.

On one level he explores how we alter a situation which we find stressful and which has the potential for crisis. To achieve this we alter the nature of the situation itself. This can involve someone altering his responses or feelings towards the stressful factor.

Alternatively, we may need to alter or deal with our thoughts in order to deal with stress. This concerns the way we manage the stress rather than altering the stressors. Some stressors become more tolerable by avoidance. Some typical and common diversions are smoking, drinking, taking drugs or overeating. These can make the stress more tolerable by avoidance, and may be our way of managing the stress.

Ask two groups to look at these two ways of coping and to give examples of their own encounters with the stress of sudden death.

The exercise should highlight how a person handles demands and conflicts, and will identify how we tolerate or minimise these. The demands and conflicts will be both from without and within. Coping will be the way we handle the feelings, thoughts and bodily responses of others.

We have said we may change the situation or manage it. There is no one way of coping with the situation. Some of it will depend on our past personal experience, personality, relationship with others and our environment. Coping is considering all of these dimensions.

How the carer sees the client as coping with sudden death may be examined in another exercise for two groups.

The feedback on the board at the front of the group

Group A	Group B
Write 10 statements: **Coping is . . .**	Write 10 statements: **Coping is not . . .**

Box 5.2 Coping is/is not.

produces food for thought on items appearing on both lists, and can provide some amusement. A little light relief is usually necessary. A common statement on both lists is:

'Coping is not crying'
and
'Coping is crying.'

A third and different exercise on coping is to discuss this statement about a close relative after a sudden death:

'What did you want the client to take away?'

This can be an exercise for two groups. For Group A add to the statement 'in the immediate care,' and for Group B 'after long-term counselling'.

This examines the expectations and goals of counselling, and should highlight our expectations about change or about allowing the client to be themselves with the carer taking on a comforting or nurturing role. We need to ask if the desired outcomes are for us or for the client.

The carer could be rejected as having nothing to offer for this particular difficulty. We may, on a personal level, be rejected. How will we respond to this? Has anyone in the helping role thought of this response as being a possibility?

WHAT INCAPACITATES US

The previous chapter has identified some of the emotional responses we are confronted with in sudden death. It will be useful to spend time looking at each one and looking at the nature of the response and the difficulties we may have with them.

These are best explored in workshops or in one day school settings. Small workshops of up to 12 people are ideal, but financially, larger groups are more viable.

I have now conducted over 100 small group workshops on coping with sudden death, and have also run larger groups. It goes without saying that working with sudden death and all its complexities demands knowledge.

It is not at all unusual to hear the statement that some people just have a gift for the work. I do not believe this, and people working with it who are well motivated do not believe it either.

They arrive on study days and at workshops with a demand to be taught the various theories on loss and the processes of grief. We have already discussed that they also need an ability to stay with pain, anguish and distress. This ability is powerful in its repercussions on the sufferer, as it validates where they are and how they feel. But this alone is not enough.

Exploring some of the responses in the previous chapter enables us to stay with these feelings and have some insight into the human response to grief.

Where this response fits in to the overall processes of the grief, and the care of the client, also becomes important. The impact of the sudden death is overwhelming and sometimes chaotic. The disorder it produces for us and for our clients can make it unmanageable. We, the carers, need to manage both the disorder and ourselves. This immediate management is reflected in the immediate or long-term coping strategies of our clients.

Using holistic care in the process of coping with crisis requires a knowledge of the skills involved. They are not magic solutions, but offer ways to make the situation manageable and to understand the nature of disordered behaviour. So teaching and training staff to work with sudden death will need some formal teaching of these theories and their application to practice.

The applications I have found useful for demonstrating on study days are found in Chapter 1, but only one or two of these need formal teaching and people need encouraging to read more about them. The usefulness of working in this way, or the constraints these structures impose upon the worker, can then be discussed in small groups. Fitting the client into the model or process of working usually produces some lively discussion .

Working with a client's life crisis requires some good inter-personal skills, as we explored earlier when talking about breaking the bad news. We need to practise these skills and to take part in exercises using listening skills, establishing eye contact and finding the right words. We need to hear our-selves say out loud words such as dying and dead.

Trying to avoid pain or distress by saying things like 'We have lost her' or 'He has slipped away' can also be checked out by doing the exercises in pairs. The words on the follow-ing list can be said out loud to another person in a pairs exercise.

Loss	Death	Coffin
Dead	Divorce	Mourning
Dying	Custody	Grave
Gone	Abandoned	Cremated
Absent	Grieving	Buried
Bereft		

Box 5.3 Words to use in exercise on communicating bad news.

As person A says the words out loud to person B, B will attempt to pick up any difficulties the speaker has from inflec-tions in the voice or from hesitations. A will be asked, whilst saying them, to try to be aware of which words cause him dif-ficulty or painful memories.

Then, without discussion, the roles are immediately reversed and B then says the words out loud to A. The same difficulties, or pain, or reluctance to use certain words, are then discussed together.

When debriefing the exercise in open discussion, issues will be raised about the rituals of death and the confrontational nature of the words. It will also have become apparent that the words in the third column are all related to ritualistic responses to death.

Other words, such as custody, divorce and separation offer a stimulus to discuss the differences, if any, between issues of death, divorce, separation and custody. This discussion should highlight the major loss experienced in these transactions, and how they may stigmatise or embarrass more than death does.

They are certainly subjects people avoid as much as death. Many people describe the anger and distress they feel when the grief of divorce is not recognised and is avoided as much as death.

It may be useful, as we look at some of the issues to be taught and explored in this chapter, if we establish some ground rules to work with. As we explore how to teach and train for this work, you may find it useful to write down the values and ways of working that it requires. The exercise just discussed, for example, requires some trust, an openness and an honesty with the person we are sharing the exercise with.

Perhaps sharing is a key to help to make it a mutually useful experience. We already have some key words for learning and working with the clients:

```
┌─────────────────────────────────────────────┐
│ Trust                                         │
│                                               │
│ Openness                                      │
│                                               │
│ Honesty                                       │
│                                               │
│ Sharing                                       │
│                                               │
│ . . . . . . .                                 │
│ . . . . . . .                                 │
└─────────────────────────────────────────────┘
```

Box 5.4 The nature of the learning — issues involved in working with sudden death — some common responses to the exercise.

The difficulty of establishing these qualities, and what they mean, can be discussed near the end of a study day when more qualities have been collected. This exercise establishes the many-faceted qualities needed for good interpersonal skills.

YOUR OWN LIFE LUGGAGE

The material you collect from your own personal experience within your family and culture can be either a hindrance or an asset. If death and its pain were denied, hidden away and not openly discussed, you may have problems working with it. You may have remained in this state of denial, or compensated so much for this, that you are at the opposite end of the spectrum. This may be perceived by some clients as being insensitive and too confronting.

It is essential therefore, that we know ourselves, understand something of the nature of our family's response to death, and acknowledge something of our cultural backgrounds. Our personal characteristics and life experiences must be examined, otherwise we will have problems if these re-emerge in a disruptive or painful way with the client.

In workshops I have conducted, many people have apologised because they have no personal experience of sudden death, or any death for that matter, in their own families. Others present sometimes suggest that it is the ultimate qualification to do the work. If you want a lively discussion, you may ask them to discuss the statement:

You only really know the pain and impact of death if you have experienced it yourself.

It will obviously produce some anxiety to use an exercise that examines our own experiences of death. The exercise should not only examine the issues involved in our 'whole life' encounter with death, but will focus on the difficulties of such an exercise. These in turn will reflect communication issues experienced daily by our clients, and will highlight how vulnerable they must feel when sharing such difficulties.

One way of looking at our own life experience and exploring its impact on us, is to use the following questionnaire (Fig. 5.1):

1. The first death I can remember was the death of:	
2. I was aged:	
3. The feelings I remember I had at the time were:	
4. The first funeral (wake or other ritual service) I ever attended was for:	
5. I was aged:	
6. The thing I most remember about that experience is :	
7. My most recent loss by death was: (person, time, circumstances)	
8. I coped with this loss by:	
9. The most difficult death for me was the death of:	
10. It was difficult because:	
11. Of the most important people in my life who are now living, the most difficult death for me would be the death of:	
12. It would be the most difficult because:	
13. My primary style of coping with loss is:	
14. I know my grief is resolved when:	
15. It is appropriate for me to share my own experience of grief with a client when:	

Figure 5.1 Questionnaire — Personal experience of death. (Reprinted from Wordon W. J. (1983) *Grief Counselling and Grief Therapy* with the kind permission of Tavistock Publications.)

Wordon (1983) lists this series of questions to help us look at our own losses. He points out that the type of client the carer will have personal difficulty with is usually related to the carer's own area of unresolved conflict.

I have 500 of these questionnaires, completed by people in caring roles — nurses, doctors, social workers, counsellors from many fields of work, voluntary workers, residential care staff and policemen. They have given me a wealth of information on some of the workers with sudden death who have participated in my workshops and study days.

I usually ask them to spend 15–20 minutes filling in the questionnaire. It will be difficult to do this too early in the session, as it is very confronting. I have found it fits in more easily at the end of the morning session, as a lunch break gives you time to leave it behind and concentrate on more formal issues.

The questions cover our life's history of confrontations with death, from childhood, to our fears for the future and our ideas on coping. The facilitator needs to remain present whilst the form is being completed, as some will need questions clarified and others may find feelings of grief re-emerge. Most people find the exercise useful as it encourages work they have not done for themselves on grief.

Some of the vulnerability that does become apparent, whilst raising anxiety or causing distress, can also be useful. If the exercise is done just prior to lunch, people will have time to pull themselves together again during the break.

Whilst the exercise is useful on a personal level, the 500 forms I have collected say a lot about what happens to people as they encounter death, both in their family and as individuals. I also wonder whether there may be some indication as to why these people in particular have ended up helping others with sudden death.

I usually break the questionnaire up into sections when discussing it later, and examine issues linked with each group of questions in turn. When the questionnaire is completed they are told this will happen, but first they are asked to pair up with someone in the room.

The exercise may be more easily facilitated if the person is a stranger to them. I often set it up so that they have carried out one previous short exercise together but before that they were strangers. I then ask them to discuss with each other:

Any issue that you have been confronted with by the questionnaire.

They are given 10 minutes only to do this. Restate the task again to make it clear what you are asking them to do. The facilitator should watch how they do this from the side of the room, and note any difficulties. Below are some behavioural signs indicating difficulty:

1. A reluctance to begin the exercise.
2. A quick completion of the exercise, avoiding eye contact or intimacy with the partner.
3. Physical closeness may be apparent, and making physical contact. Giving each other good attention.
4. Being embarrassed at obvious distress, or responding to it comfortably.
5. Looking around the room uncomfortably, observing whether others are able to take part in the exercise.
6. Tight lipped and rigid demeanour, throwing hostile glances towards the facilitator. Resentment at the exercise is apparent.
7. When told it is time to stop, how long does it take them to disengage from the interaction?

Some of these observations you may make known to the group after they have examined the exercise all together. In debriefing the exercise, remind them of the task of the encounter, i.e. to discuss any issue you have been confronted with by the questionnaire.

Ask them to help you make a list of the difficulties in doing this. It is essential they stick to the task of the debrief, i.e. to examine the difficulties of that 10-minute interaction and the difficulties of the questionnaire. The difficulties usually listed are:

```
Makes you feel vulnerable
Unresolved loss re-emerges
Difficulty controlling emotions
Resentment/anger at being asked
  to reveal personal material
Finding the right words
Time constraint
Lack of privacy
Is it easier with a stranger?
```

Box 5.5 Difficulties of the task — some common responses to the exercise.

Remind them that, in our interactions with clients, the clients experience all these difficulties. This is what it feels like to be asked to share feelings of grief and loss.

We can become blasé and insensitive about inviting people to share pain and distress, and it is, in fact, an awkward thing to do. Have we forgotten how embarrassing and vulnerable the client can feel when sharing pain and distress? The exercise is to remind us that we too can be clients, and this is how it feels to be one.

Another issue worth discussing is what conditions or surroundings do we offer people to talk in. Lack of privacy, feelings emerging where others are present or overhearing, may be discussed in debriefing this exercise. Many hospitals are very poor at providing areas where people can hear bad news with privacy.

Distressed people have been told of someone's sudden death in a corridor where they were overheard, or where many people were passing. Others described sitting in an office where people interrupted to answer telephones or collect materials.

The exercise highlights how it feels to share sensitive things in public or exposed surroundings. The value of providing private rooms and facilities for the suddenly bereaved needs more attention. Clients may later become fixed on difficulties linked with this.

This exercise usually takes 15–20 minutes to debrief. You will need to make participants focus on the interaction and not the content of the questionnaire.

EXAMINING THE QUESTIONNAIRE ON ENCOUNTERING DEATH

Breaking down the questionnaire usually produces some lively discussions, and particular issues are linked with separate sets of questions. It always amazes me how participants are willing to share personal encounters with death. They can be relied upon to highlight differences and how the differences are perceived.

Some people clearly believe that their family's experience of and response to death was healthy and useful. Others will say the opposite. Begin by examining questions 1–6.

Questions 1–6

This usually produces issues of children, childhood and family responses to death. Discussion about the age at which children understand about the concept of death and its meaning produces lots of anecdotes.

A common source of anger, and one apparent in my 500 questionnaires, concerns grandparents. There must be hundreds of adults walking around angry and resentful at being excluded from a grandparent's funeral as a child. Many describe returning home from school to discover relatives in the house and the funeral over. Others learnt of the death from a person other than a parent, and are angry that parents were unable or failed to tell them.

This discussion inevitably leads on to the community's response to death. Older people will describe relatives lying in a coffin in the 'front room' and the ritual drawing of the curtains. All the neighbours, and the community, could see the clear signs of a death. Others will describe how, nowadays, there are few signs of death and people discover a neighbour has died many weeks after the event.

The discussion arising from the first six questions raises many issues concerning children, families, and communal responses to death. In debriefing the questionnaire, it is a fairly safe place to begin.

Questions 7–10

I use the discussion of our recent actual encounters with death to examine some of the stresses of working with sudden death. It may be useful to present questions about the difficulty of separating our losses from our work. You may pose a problem, such as 'How do you work with the death of someone's mother or father, when you have just experienced the death of your own?'

Discussion on separating our own grief from the client's, and focusing on our own needs, is usually animated. I am constantly reminded in these discussions how we ask for very little for ourselves. Somehow it is seen as self-indulgence, and the carer's expectations of themselves are outrageous.

We do not demand from our clients what we demand from ourselves. Someone will always describe going back to work after the statutory 3 days compassionate leave, and expecting themselves or being expected to become re-immersed in caring for the bereaved immediately. Anxiety is always expressed that to state this is difficult, or to ask for help is a sign of weakness, or that it will be recorded against them.

Another problem is that there are few or no resources within the system to care for or counsel the staff. Ask the group why, when you begin to discuss the needs and difficulties stemming from the staff's personal encounters with death, they become quiet. Ask why it is difficult for them to talk about their own needs. Does it say something about the carers, that with other people's difficulties they feel needed or powerful or in a position of strength, but are unwilling to deal with their own needs?

Discussion of the personality profiles of carers rarely fails to provoke responses.

Questions 11–12

Half the people present will have failed to answer the questions honestly. Many will have refused to answer them and simply have put a line through them. Others will have put someone's name down and crossed it out. Trying to be honest in answering these two questions will produce guilt and conflict. There will be very few who are comfortable with and are clear about their answer.

Question 11 asks them to name **one** person. Few will have been able to do this. Those who are mothers of more than one child will say it is impossible to say one child's loss would be more difficult than another's.

I would refute that. Many parents whom I have seen for long-term counselling have needed to discuss difficulties with their grief, because one child's death is commonly more difficult than another's, since our relationships with each of our children are unique and valued for different reasons.

With adults, one person's death could also be more difficult than another's. Some participants will reject this because they do not want to explore it. If we are going to work with sudden death at its onset or later, we must be aware of our own worst fears.

When we are confronted with these fears in others, and particularly if we have to work with them, we need to have some insight into why the work may be especially difficult. When we are confronted with our own worst fears in our clients, we are likely to be less effective and consequently to struggle with the work.

The difficulty will be even worse if we deny the connection of being confronted with our own worst fears. If we acknowledge this difficulty we will find some way of compensating for it. More than that, we will forgive ourselves for finding the interaction difficult. We will then have some insight into how our fears can make us less effective.

In an earlier case study, where a nurse refused to acknowledge this with the result that she rushed a lady out before she was ready to go back home, the nurse had been confronted with her own worst fears. If she had acknowledged this it would have been less powerful. The client was clearly aware of the nurse's difficulty, and later remarked on it:

'She must have had a husband the same age as mine. She could not cope with me.'

Question 12, on why it would be difficult, I do not pursue in the workshop setting. The issues in this are acknowledged in Question 11, and must remain with the individual for the moment.

Questions 13 and 14

This can be a short discussion on how our views on coping can vary. Another exercise — What is coping? — is described on page 116.

The word 'resolved' in Question 14 is most useful. It highlights issues of grief, and inevitably this leads to discussion on resolution being too high an expectation. The question then arises — Is grief ever resolved? It becomes important in training sessions to identify how one word can produce so much material from the group.

Question 15

Discuss here how the experience of grief is a unique and individual experience. It is easy to dilute someone else's experience or distract or divert them from it to your own. That may suit us if we are having difficulty with the client's pain.

Many people will describe how you can make use of your own experience in a constructive and sensible way.

One suggested rule about this is to offer only your own material if asked to. I have rarely been asked at the impact of loss, and would certainly not offer it at this time. In long-term counselling, clients often need a glimpse of the person behind the role of counsellor. They often ask the counsellor to reveal vulnerability about themselves. In this situation it seems more appropriate.

The whole exercise using this questionnaire should be given a total time of 1½ hours. It can certainly be given no less. At the end, stress how the deaths we have experienced fit into a whole life experience. Describe the journey you have made together — perhaps from childhood to present losses and on to fears of future losses — and how we might feel coping with all this.

The exercise is difficult, and people should be thanked for taking part and encountering a sometimes painful glimpse of themselves. Remind them how we expect clients to do this.

It is worth saying that it is not at all unusual for unresolved difficulties to emerge, and if people are to be effective in this work the difficulties may require further time and attention. They may need to find someone — a friend or colleague — to talk to. This exercise is essential for people involved in long-term counselling. You may find it useful to fill in the questionnaire for yourself, now.

Although it is the subject of the next chapter, many of the questions on this list offer the worker a chance to examine personal difficulties. The problem can be who has been available to help with them.

BEHAVIOUR AND FEELINGS CONNECTED WITH LOSS

How we feel and behave when we discover the loss of something we value reflects some of the overall difficulties in sudden death.

An exercise that looks at this but also encourages course participants to meet and talk to each other is the searching game.

Everyone is asked to pair up with someone in the room they

do not know. After a few minutes spent introducing themselves to each other they begin the exercise. Try to encourage them to sit facing each other and put down any papers, so they can give each other plenty of attention.

They are asked to spend 3 minutes each describing how they felt on discovering the loss of some object that they have valued. It must not be a person or a living thing such as a pet. As well as how they felt on discovering the loss, they are asked to say how they set about finding the object. The person listening is asked to help her partner share his feelings about the loss.

At the end of 3 minutes call time, and then ask the other person to describe the object she lost. It may help the group to remember some incident if you remind them that it may have been something that was borrowed and never returned, or something stolen, or something lost through carelessness.

After the total 6 minutes, ask the group to look to the front and make two lists on the board. One will be headed 'feelings', and the other 'behaviour'.

Begin with the list headed 'feelings' by asking them to describe how they felt on discovering the loss. Below is a typical response, with the words that will stimulate discussion.

Anger directed at self
Anger directed at others
Denial
Sadness
Panic
Regret
Acceptance
Resignation
Confusion
Fear
Anxiety
Resentment
Suspicion
Hope

Box 5.6 Feelings on discovering the loss — some common responses to the exercise.

These words will all help to stimulate discussion.

You should then ask how they set about finding the object. Here is a list of typical responses:

Panic/disorder/chaos
Searching — disordered
            — more orderly
Retracing steps
Compulsive/obsessive behaviour
Concealment
Intense activity
Inactivity (resignation)
Enlisting help
Replacing
Diversions
Defensive (bolts, padlocks etc.)

Box 5.7 Behaviour on discovering the loss — some common responses to the exercise.

Again, with the words on the list, there is plenty to stimulate discussion. Remind them, on looking at the two lists, that this is a glimpse of themselves and their responses to losses.

Ask them which of the feelings and behaviour they are more accepting of within themselves or others. Ask them which behaviour or feelings they become angry with, or find unacceptable. This will help to identify some feelings and responses we have an inbuilt difficulty with.

Return to both lists and ask people to think about them in response to sudden death. They will be able to identify responses on the list with suddenly bereaved people they have met.

Some of these responses the carer will find more manageable, others will be very distressing and difficult to respond to. It will become apparent as you explore the responses that the intense, disordered or chaotic behaviour will be more difficult for the carer, the client, his family and friends to tolerate.

The feelings, although painful, will somehow seem easier for the carer to respond to. The behaviour adds to the feelings of disorder, loss of control, and the potential for madness. It is little wonder that we will have greater problems in coping with this on a personal, professional and skills level.

The whole exercise, exploring all the aspects discussed, can take 1–2 hours. Shortened versions may be used by presenting the direct relationship with sudden death but making the connection later, when discussing behaviour in a crisis or when looking at the crisis process.

SILENCES

As this was identified in the previous chapter as something that makes us feel uncomfortable, this exercise allows us to stay with and identify feelings without verbalising them. Again this exercise is carried out in pairs. Each person has to take some stance that describes a feeling, e.g. withdrawal, agitation, perplexity.

Ask participants to think of some of the feelings on discovering a loss from the previous exercise. Person A acts out non-verbally the feeling and B mirrors this. These can be in the standing or sitting position. B should make every effort to mirror A exactly, taking particular note of the position of the head, limbs, feet and distribution of weight.

After A has spent 5 minutes initiating the non-verbalised feelings it is then B's turn.

At the end of this, ask them how they felt about their closeness to the other person's feelings. Which one could they emulate most easily and feel the closest to, and which left them feeling uncomfortable.

Another exercise to examine the difficulty of silence is to spend 2 minutes in three different postures, in silence:

1. Back to back
2. Side by side
3. Facing each other with knees touching.

They should discuss what they learnt about themselves and others by doing this.

Whilst the exercises concerning silences have much to teach us, they can also be fun. This is a necessary ingredient in a day dealing with sudden death.

REFLECTING FEELINGS

We have already identified that it is easier to work with the feelings behind the behaviour. Difficult and disordered behaviour causes distress for the carer as well as for the client. The shift to the feelings underlying the behaviour helps to put some order and meaning into the situation, and explains some of the disorder.

Again, participants are split up into pairs. A talks to B about an incident which produced lots of feelings. If people need help with this, suggest something from childhood, or a holiday incident which perhaps produced anxiety as well as pleasure.

A talks for 4 minutes about this incident. B then reflects the feelings but not the content. Allow 2 minutes for this and then reverse the process.

This should help with focusing on feelings and practising putting them into words.

OPPOSITE ENDS OF THE SPECTRUM

This exercise is another way of gaining a wider vocabulary on feelings which will help us to find a range of words that describe the client's feelings. Sometimes, when working with the grieving process, it helps us if we evaluate where the client has arrived at.

In this situation, we need to allow ourselves to be wrong, to have used the wrong word to describe how they are feeling and to be able to say:

'I see, do you mean . . .?'

and then offer another word. This exercise gives practice in identifying and describing feelings.

Draw a line down the middle of a sheet of paper and put two words that describe opposite extremes (Fig. 5.2), one at the top and the other at the bottom.

Now write down words in between that describe feelings along this spectrum. Try other moods with variations, such as Irritation to Rage.

After spending 5 minutes on two ranges of words, work in small groups to share the difficulties and the words you find useful or apt for situations. Ask participants to discuss how some words describe such extreme distress and are so powerful that we are reluctant to use them.

The exercise should help us to gain a wider vocabulary to describe feelings, and become more sensitive to the level of feelings that people have arrived at.

A variation on the exercise is to look at the line and the words at the top and bottom. Begin in the middle by describ-

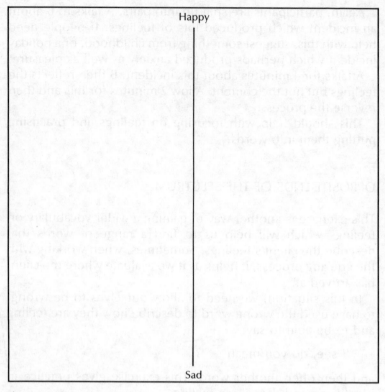

Figure 5.2 Opposite extremes.

ing a situation and take it to an extreme. This should highlight how people often begin somewhere safe and how we can take them sensitively to some of the more powerful feelings and difficulties.

In looking at the communication issues in sudden death, both in the immediate or long term, we have looked at our attempts to communicate meaningfully, using words that convey how people are feeling, and where they move up and down the spectrum of those feelings. Whilst this may make us more effective in our communications, there are qualities that people will want to see and experience in us that help them to be comfortable with our persona. An exercise to help us explore this I will call:

Someone I like talking to

Ask the group to spend 5 minutes thinking about a friend or

colleague to whom they would not mind talking if they had some difficulty or something good to share. Ask them to make a list of the qualities in that person which make him or her special, e.g.:

Accessible
Good listener
Non-judgemental
Unlimited time
Comforting
Friendship
. . . . .
. . . . .
. . . . .
. . . . .

Box 5.8 List of qualities — some common responses to the exercise.

When they have made the list, write some of these qualities on the board. When the list is completed, ask them as a group which qualities you can tick that apply to the client/counsellor relationship.

This should provide some good discussion when, for example, you arrive at qualities such as open accessibility or friendship. This leads on to the degree of intimacy of the relationship, and issues about separating it from one's personal life.

Allow 30 minutes to discuss these difficulties. Any stronger, more difficult problems can be given back to two smaller groups to explore in more detail. These discussions need only last 10–15 minutes.

Body talk

What your body says about you is not always apparent to you. We all pick up habits that are irritating or do not convey what we are trying to say. For example, we may tap our foot if irritated or feel someone is being long-winded in his explanation of something.

Is the foot tapping an expression of our irritation, or something we do when we have difficulty concentrating? If it is the latter this is our problem and it should not be conveyed in this way.

Two- or three-day training sessions may allow us to explore in more detail some of these communication issues. When people have had the opportunity to achieve a rapport with fellow workers on a workshop you may, as a trainer, consider this exercise to explore non-verbal communication:

Posture	
Breathing	
Voice	
Face	
Eyes	
Mannerisms	
Time response	
Anything else significant	

Figure 5.3 My body talk.

There are two ways you can use this form. The first is to use your own awareness to explore the issues involved in each section, and record how you see your strengths and weaknesses. Some sections you may not have considered, and may give them some thought as you work on the training issues.

An exercise to use over the period of a day or two, especially for people working in pairs, is to ask the other person to make some observations about you in each section, over a longer period, and then evaluate the exercise towards the end of a training session. The observations made can be both positive and negative. This is not meant to be a demoralising experience.

This is by no means a definitive way of looking at each section, but some people may need help with their approach to it. One of the problems of training for this kind of work is that the participants attending the course will have differing amounts of experience and training. Some questions that may help you to explore each section are as follows.

Posture

Do you slouch down in the chair?
Do you sit huddled and appear motionless to pain and anguish?
Does this imply to the client that this is damaging you?
Do you sit with arms folded?

Breathing

What do your deep sighs mean to others?
Is the way you are breathing a sign of your tension or difficulty with this client or with the material?

Voice

Listen for changes in tone or strength.
At what pace do words emerge?
Is there some pressure of speech?
Do regional accents matter?
In our attempts to reassure, is our tone patronising?

Face

Do we have one expression for the whole time?

Does our expression convey what we mean?

Do we smile? Beware of the fixed smile, particularly if accompanied by the 'there there, it will be all right' words.

Mouth and jaw held rigid may indicate tension and anxiety.

Eyes

Do we avoid eye contact?

How do we fix our eyes, and remain attentive and relaxed?

Are some stares intrusive?

Do we know when to look away?

Avoid gazing around the room as though uninterested.

Mannerisms

Your use of hands and body movements may give life and meaning to what you say. Constantly picking something up and putting it down, or dismantling a pen, may irritate, especially if you drop the parts and have to search round for them, or cannot fix it together again.

Some mannerisms are your hallmark, or say a lot about you, and are not necessarily negative. You may have a certain way you straighten your hair or rest your head on your hands.

Time response

Do you hear things out, or terminate other people's conversation prematurely?

Are you able to use your time to give structure to your counselling? Are you able to begin it and take it to an appropriate end?

Does an awareness of time elapsing produce other body talk?

Anything else of significance?

Some people may want to discuss other issues here which they feel can cause a distraction from the counselling or a difficulty in rapport. Will that ring through your nose be off-putting to the client? A discussion on prejudice, and how it is dealt with, may result.

In looking specifically at counselling or communication skills for the suddenly bereaved, this exercise may appear to deal with a peripheral issue, but in longer sessions of training, these other aspects of counselling skills offer some light relief and help people relax. The ability to use the knowledge, and communicate effectively, is very important.

SETTING UP STUDY DAYS AND WORKSHOPS

Whilst some space is necessary for what people bring, some structure removes anxiety. The exercises or approaches discussed offer some ways of exploring the issues involved in sudden death, and a way of teaching some skills and theory connected with it.

In a small workshop group, they can be made available and introduced after a joint decision on how to use the day. Most people are more comfortable with some clear direction or structure to work within and larger groups are much more manageable if the day is organised.

A programme sent out prior to the day will also mean delegates will have given some thought to the ideas before the event.

The planned use of the personal material of the helpers, or their experiences, in exercises, should be stated explicitly on the programme. The use of experiential exercises, as well as a straightforward look at the theory, must be made clear prior to the day.

People then put themselves there voluntarily, and know what may be expected of them, and that their input is vital to the success of the day. They can, of course, opt out, and the facilitator must be sensitive to people's difficulties and have the resources to deal with them. Most difficulties can be used to reflect the concerns and problems of us all and can allow people the opportunity to care for and support colleagues.

When teaching and training people to work with sudden death, the pain and problems of the helper will become apparent. This cannot be avoided. All we have to try to ensure is that the carers themselves will be cared for, not only by us in our training but also within the structure of our organisations.

Teaching and training will require sensitivity to the carers' distress. It will also become apparent that, when this emerges, some workers cannot cope with or tolerate vulnerability in each other.

We are vulnerable, there is no doubt about that, and colleagues can respond to our vulnerability in a way which does not indicate that we are unsuitable, or less of a person, for this becoming apparent.

When this happens on workshops you arrange, you may be accused of letting it happen or not preventing it (not quite the same thing). You may be accused of introducing material that is too personal and creeps through carers' defences and causes some stress.

Clients have a way of doing just that.

Working with sudden death is stressful. We must now consider how to manage this stress.

REFERENCES

Lazarus R 1966 Psychological stress and the coping process. McGraw Hill, New York

Wordon J W 1983 Grief counselling and grief therapy. Tavistock, London

6

The stress of caring

There is no way of working through the intervention skills needed in sudden death, without arriving here at the stress of it all. I hope that the way we have looked at each aspect of sudden death helps you to arrive at this point better armed to deal with the stress.

In Chapter 1 we looked at some structured ways of working with sudden death. Crisis intervention, a holistic approach or whatever structure we use can help to put some order into a chaotic, disordered episode of life. This is one way to deal with some of the stress. It certainly helps me to structure my thoughts more usefully when there is pain and disorder around me.

We then moved on to looking at the immediate needs of the family. This opportunity to facilitate their search for resources takes some effort and concentration on the part of the carer. In our immediate care of the family we may simply be in a nurturing role, providing care and safety. This giving, this caring, may make us feel useful and at the time may dissipate any stress we feel.

As we moved on to the long-term implications of the care, we gained, I hope, some insight into the value of what we do. This is just what we need when we suffer doing the job.

In preparing ourselves for the stress, we looked at responses that incapacitate us, and doing this should remove some of the perplexity or difficulty of being confronted with these responses. This leads on to being educated and trained for the work, and how we might be taught effectively. Armed with some knowledge we feel less defenceless.

By reading more widely — and the books listed in the bibliography may help here — we will gain greater insight into the mechanisms, both physical and psychological, that emerge at an encounter with sudden death. This insight will remove some of the mystery of the nature of people's responses.

Ideally, in our search for knowledge about working with sudden death, we have learned that whatever way people respond, it is a valid response for them. There is no right or wrong about it, and we must not judge them.

In theory, then, we should have arrived at a position of strength. There is, however, a problem with all this and we have already discussed it. These thoughts, theories and structures to work with are for the clients. They are not for us. We have different values for ourselves:

Ann was recognised within her Emergency Department as having a caring manner when dealing with relatives. Whilst she had to have all the skills of a critical care nurse, her particular forté was caring for distressed relatives and the emotional distress in the patient.

Over the years she had gained so much from these people, both in knowledge and in an increase in her own skills. If she knew some members of staff had difficulty with this, she would offer to take work from them, or talk to them afterwards about how they coped and what they had learned.

She often reflected on how she walked into outrageously painful situations and attempted to begin something useful, and what it was doing to her. She felt she had something to give and to gain.

For the past 6 months, however, she felt that this had altered. She seemed to be giving more than she gained. There were times when she resented being asked for help by other members of staff, but this was natural, she thought.

Recently it had been worse than this — worse because her response was more extreme and worse because she did not realise what was happening. At least previously she had thought her resentment a natural response. Now she had no idea that her response was anger, accusation and bitterness.

Some days it was painfully apparent. When a friend and colleague could not cope with the parents of a teenager dying from a motor cycle accident, she had had some advice and suggestions to offer her:

'Perhaps you are in the wrong job. If you can't stand the heat, why are you here? You are no use to them like this. You have to be strong. If you are after promotion it will not look very good for you.'

These words were coming from Ann — Ann who was usually so outspoken when others responded in this way. Resentfully, she went to care for these people and in her anger and sure knowledge of what they wanted, failed to hear what they were saying to her. She had a recipe of skills that would suit their every need, and she forgot how defenceless and at the mercy of others, people in this position were.

A few days later she was complaining how tired she felt, and how the job was playing havoc with her back, and the rushed meals were giving her indigestion. Her monologue was interrupted by a man shouting in the next room.

She knew he was the man whose daughter had taken an overdose, and who was complaining at the length of time she had been kept waiting for treatment.

Ann immediately bemoaned the fact that staff nowadays were so young and inexperienced and not firm enough with people: these people need to be kept in their place, who do they think they are? After all, the girl brought this on herself. The father was probably feeling guilty about not caring for his daughter properly. Ann had not met the man or his daughter, but she immediately knew what it was about.

Two weeks later during the coffee break, a tired-looking Ann told the whole staff room how much the job had changed. People were too well cared for these days. They expect you to do everything for them. We cannot go on giving more and more without more help. Ann went on to say how people at the top had no idea about what was going on.

A few days later she was again late coming off duty. She decided it was better to sort out the complicated things yourself, in case it all went wrong. You are only left to sort out a mess, she thought. The trouble is, you cannot trust other people to do it.

As she drove home to her flat, where she lived alone, she thought of the little old lady whose husband had suddenly dropped down dead that day, and who would be at home, alone. Suddenly, Ann began to cry for her and for herself. All the cars hooting reminded her that the lights had turned to green, and she mouthed a rude comment to the nearest driver.

'What's happening to me?' she thought. 'My mother would be horrified at what I have just said. It's this city, it's the job. I just need a holiday.'

She rang in the following day, to say she was ill with a migraine. She was irritated because the receiver of the call had remarked that Ann was getting lots of short periods of illness. The next day she was not well, but went to work because she felt guilty. Within a few hours she felt quite bright and engrossed in some routine, straightforward tasks like doing dressings and bandages — nothing too demanding.

A call came from ambulance control. A mother and child were being brought from a house fire. Neither was breathing.

Ann felt panic. Why didn't this happen yesterday? Why does it always happen when I'm here? I have had too many of these bad ones to deal with. I wish I could just run away, she thought.

Her thoughts were interrupted by a voice saying:

'Ann, the police have just rung. They have found the husband/father of the house fire victims at work. They are bringing him in now. Do you want to speak to him?'

STRESS

Before we consider the plight of this particular helper, we should consider what we mean by stress. Stress is not necessarily a bad thing, and the word is often used with strong negative connotations when in fact stress can be very useful.

Stress is a message that some coping is required. It is a signal to mobilise some resources. As discussed in Chapter 5 on training, stress is about excessive internal and external demands and our response to these. What is stressful depends on the way we think about ourselves, and the situation we are in. We then have to consider the demands being made upon us, and what these demands mean.

Although we may value the importance of caring for others, there may be a cost to us personally. How we manage these demands depends on our tolerance to what we are confronted with, and whether or not we have any control or mastery over the situation.

If we can reduce or minimise the disorder in the situation, some order or control will result. Control is a word used often in training sessions, for coping is not necessarily about success but about change and our efforts to manage or control it. The outcome may not be what we want, but we may be satisfied with our input in order to alter it, or we may adapt to it.

So stress may be the mechanism through which we find ways of coping with something difficult.

IDENTIFICATION

For most people, an encounter with a death that intimately concerns them occurs only a few times in their lives. Some people will talk of hearing of several deaths recently, but these may have no profound implications for them. They merely know them or of them.

Working with sudden death means one encounter after another, and may mean an intimate knowledge of its effect on loved ones. The carer will often ask herself what effect this abnormal exposure to death is having upon her. Other people will ask her how she copes with it all, some hoping to hear of some secret formula that protects her from it.

One of the mechanisms for the carer to explore is that of identification. We sometimes talk of putting ourselves in another person's place to try to imagine what her needs are and to increase our sensitivity.

If we do not have the ability to disengage from it and to remember that:

I am not you and the feelings are yours not mine

we are in trouble. We can become burdened with emotion

that does not belong to us and become less effective as a carer.

Identification may occur because of similar life styles, sex, age, occupation or appearance of the client. The identification then becomes a mechanism by which the carer patterns his personality on that of the client, assuming that person's qualities, characteristics and responses.

We need to be constantly sensitive to this possibility occurring.

DISPLACEMENT

This mechanism can also result in stress, and can add to the burden of the carer unless he has some insights into it. We have considered displacement earlier when exploring the issue of advocacy in health care settings. The response of:

> 'How can you ask her to see the body, you are adding to her distress'

was one example of this. A more accurate response would be:

> 'Asking her to do that will distress her and add to my distress, and I will be left to pick up the pieces.'

Displacement is the shift of an emotion from the person it was directed towards, to another person (or object), usually neutral or less dangerous. This mechanism is not only a difficulty on impact of sudden death, but often arises in bereavement counselling.

Carers need to be aware of the difference between displacement and projection. Projection is when the client attributes his own thoughts or impulses to another person. When this other person is always the carer, the carer can find it very stressful. This is particularly so if there is marked anger or aggression.

Some examples:

'At the hospital, at the time of a sudden death, I was discussing with the deceased's companion the handing over of valuables and jewellery. She became very angry and accused me of suggesting that she was immediately going to gain from

his death. This was her response when I told her I could not hand over a large sum of money found on the patient since she had informed me she was not a relative.

She said the money was hers, and despite my saying I was not refuting that but needed evidence, and that I had to go through the correct procedures, more projections occurred. She went on to say that I thought she only cared for this man to extract money from him, that I thought she was cold blooded and criminal.

In a powerful outpouring of emotion, it became apparent that these were also the thoughts of some of his relatives. I had no reason at all to suspect her motives, and was only trying to explain the intricacies of the procedure for handing over money.

Another lady, whose husband died after throwing himself from a tall building, said to me shortly after she was told of his death:

"You think I drove him to it, don't you? I have no-one else if that's what you think. I don't suppose you have ever got it wrong, said the wrong thing and regretted it. All right, you think I'm a bitch."' '

All this anger and bitterness can make the carer, against whom it is directed, feel very defensive and vulnerable. This causes even more problems. The defensiveness can be interpreted as confirmation that you do indeed feel how they thought you did, when nothing could be further from the truth.

If your response is 'Why do you think that?,' the projection may then be generalised and made less personal:

'That's what people will think, I know.'

Generalisations may be more easily worked with as the carer may be more comfortable with them, and will find them less confronting.

It is obviously useful, then, to have some knowledge of these mechanisms, these common responses to acute distress. They are then mostly understood by and acceptable to the carer.

On some days, however, we may feel a little more vulnerable, and may have lost this insight. Somewhere along our own life's experience, we may find this displacement painful, accusatory, judgemental, and can suddenly feel ineffectual, and perhaps angry.

A colleague may remind us, when we feel like this, what the response was about.

THE COST OF CARING

The cost of caring may be expressed both emotionally and physically. Because of the nature of the work, the caregivers may themselves becomes the casualties.

Bailey (1985), in his evaluation of the research in this field as well as his own, would say that nurses and doctors are more at risk than those they care for. He cites how this group, and other allied health professionals, are more exactingly exposed to greater suffering.

Allied to this exposure are other issues involved in sudden death; issues arising in immediate care but which will re-emerge for counsellors of the suddenly bereaved.

Ethical issues about resuscitation measures being discontinued are usually straightforward. You may feel that, in these situations, nothing ever is, but occasionally team members disagree on the timing of cessation of attempts. Most teams consult all members and reach an agreement.

Melia (1987) discusses how the power usually lies with the doctors, but how nurses have to put that decision into practice with or without them. This may mean deciding to no longer respond to and intervene with cardiac arrhythmias, or turning off the oxygen supply.

Melia describes how, for the nurse, the main concern may be about issues of power or control. Nurses working in critical care will be well aware of being surrounded by people and activity, only to be left alone with a bloody and broken body when all this activity has ceased.

Julie had worked in Emergency for 3 years. Despite its demands and difficulties, she got something from its variety and unpredictability.

It was a usual Saturday night with its quota of road traffic accidents and victims of assault and crime. The patients and friends were noisy, and at times disruptive. Julie had grown to be quite comfortable with this.

She was summoned to the resuscitation room where a 17-year-old youth had arrived with two stab wounds to the abdomen. He was shocked, gasping for breath, and had classical signs of air hunger.

There were a lot of people in the room, all making demands. Intravenous lines were quickly established, blood sent to the lab for group- and cross-matching, cardiac monitoring begun and a central venous line established. Continuous blood pressure and pulse monitoring indicated a fast-deteriorating condition. He was bleeding to death despite vigorous efforts to save him.

People were becoming impatient with each other, some were beginning to shout if instruments or equipment did not just suddenly appear. Fear and frustration at losing the fight to save him were being expressed in this way.

The decision was made to do an emergency laparotomy. His abdomen was opened and the enormity of his wounds became apparent — severe damage to the arteries and liver.

Finding this, in the blood-filled cavity of the abdomen, took some time. Time he did not have. The patient was by now ventilated and having external cardiac massage. Shouts for more of this and that were heard, but it was too late.

The patient was dead and a decision to abandon the resuscitation was made. The patient's abdomen was sewn up, he was disconnected from the monitors, and the intubation tubes removed. The hissing of the oxygen ceased, as did the suctions. The high activity came to a halt, and several people left the room.

Julie looked at her colleague, then at the still, lifeless body waiting to be washed. The room was quiet.

'This is the end of the line,' Julie thought. 'This is what you are left with when you don't succeed, and when people fight and kill each other.'

Julie said to her friend:

'Do we know who he is? We don't even have a name. I wonder if his Mum and Dad are waiting for him to come home.'

As they washed his damaged young body, they both unashamedly cried.

At times, we are left powerless and helpless. Little wonder then, that we can be left with physical and emotional burdens that are too much to bear, and the cost of caring results in burnout.

BURNOUT

Burnout, in the caring or helping professions, can be viewed or defined in various ways. If we begin with the client's perspective, he sees or experiences someone who is no longer committed, lacks the energy for the work, or fails to see any useful outcome. From the client's point of view, there is a lack of care in them, or in the job.

From the carer's point of view it may be that the complete reverse of this has produced the burnout. Over-commitment, over-concern, over-investment of energy and resources has left little for self. The loss of idealism, purpose and energy, which is so necessary and seen as so vital in caring for the bereaved, is a cause for grief.

The carers themselves become overwhelmed with sadness for the predicament they are in, and may well display all those emotional responses we talked of in the client in Chapter 4. Anger, denial, crying and withdrawal may well be overt symptoms in our burnout professional.

Because we may want to deny that we are as vulnerable as our clients, our intervention may be late or difficult. You may feel that we cannot stay with our own vulnerability because to do so may make us so aware of our own fragility that we would be unable to function effectively.

Nevertheless we must not be so well defended that we fail to care for ourselves. It is not inevitable that working with sudden death will produce burnout. If we need to be defended enough to work effectively with it, and I am not sure we do, we must have some mechanism whereby our colleagues are able to respond to us, and intervene at the appropriate time, i.e. before we feel damaged.

Where burnout is present, it will be expressed in various physical and emotional forms.

Physical signs of burnout

Fatigue, loss of energy and drive, feelings of weariness and exhaustion.

Coughs, colds, headaches that take a long time to clear up.
Nausea, indigestion, colicky pain, diarrhoea, constipation.
Disturbed sleep, waking tired.
'Working all night in our dreams.'
Difficulty getting off to sleep or waking early.
Suddenly waking remembering some incident at work, or something we have forgotten to do.
Itching, rashes, dry or oily skin.
Shortness of breath or hyperventilating with tachycardia.
Wheezing.
General malaise, aches and pains, unexplained loss of energy.

There is usually perplexity and preoccupation with the above, and an underlying anxiety that you may have some serious, debilitating illness. Lots of time can be spent pondering over the nature of the illness and discussing its outcome.

Emotional

Emotionally labile, i.e. oversensitive, irritable, easily moved to tears and marked distress.
Quickly in touch with anger, or moved from irritability to anger. A need to blame others, or point the finger.
Surprise at the sudden emergence of this anger with apparently little justified stimulus. An inappropriateness about it.
Strong feelings of sadness or hopelessness. This might take on a global aspect, such as being fearful for mankind and its inhumanity or self-destructiveness.
Outbursts of screaming and shouting. Lashing out.
Suspicion that easily becomes overt paranoia. Thoughts that people are talking about you, particularly to do with your effectiveness or lack of control. This leads to thoughts of going mad.
Avoiding clients/patients and commitments to caring for them.
Finding trivial reasons for not encountering them.
Becoming bogged down in paperwork or bureaucracy.
Difficulty concentrating, or not wanting to. Lack of energy, lethargy. Difficulty staying with the focus.

One counsellor's story

'Work is one long struggle. At our place it's a constant struggle to keep in with the boss and keep enough credibility for her deputy's job, which will soon become vacant. She's the lucky one, leaving soon.

I get fed up with teaching new staff and dealing with the endless number of people doing research into this and that, and asking questions. Soon it will be school-kids for work experience. As if we didn't have enough to do. Someone is always coming up with something new, some idea to streamline or improve the organisation. It is all a constant change and a hassle.

I want to be left alone just to get on with my own work. I'm not sure if I like it any more.'

Responses to signs of burnout

Naturally, it is not enough just to know what burnout is. We should also know what can be done about it. Having decided that working with sudden death is beginning to overwhelm you, here are some suggestions that may afford some help: the anxiety is that there may be some cost to remedying the problem.

There is not only a cost to caring, but a cost to the remedy. The answer to preventing yourself further pain or distress may demand some change that is frightening. When the dissatisfaction is removed, we need to be sure we want what is left, or that we can move in a direction that offers something new and satisfying.

Sometimes, one of the problems for nurses working in critical care areas is that they cannot cope with the deaths. This particularly applies to young people dying. These critical care areas also have lots of technology, excessive demands for beds, often poor resources and staff shortages.

Manley (1986), an intensive care nurse teacher, identified workload and environment as major stressors for intensive care nurses. Next were emotional issues relating to death and severe illness. Following on from these two were inter-staff stress and responsibility for life and death decisions.

Pot-Mees (1987), in discussing the stress in Bone Marrow

Transplant Units, describes how the holistic approach to nursing care, whilst having its rewards, means a closer encounter with the relatives' fears, frustrations and anger as well as the rewards of seeing patients recover.

This new and challenging role means the nurse is more vulnerable and is subject to more stress than in the past. The ability to work with high technology and more concrete issues, and then having to make a shift to working with someone's feelings, is not an easy transition to make. This article recognises the difficulty and personal risk of working in this holistic way. It also says this is possible with good support systems, outside distractions and personal insight.

Working with the immediate issues of sudden death in hospitals is possible over a long period of time if we maintain a personal belief in ourselves and our effectiveness in this situation, if we believe in the strength, resources and resilience of people, and have good support systems.

If we are having difficulty with these, we may consider the following options:

1. Re-education or further education

Depending on where we are working with sudden death, i.e. in the immediate or the long term, we need some affirmation of the whole spectrum of it. If we only work with its immediate effects we need to have the long-term value of the work reaffirmed. Most people find resources to handle a sudden bereavement, and we may need evidence of this.

If we work with the long term, we need to know that people do progress from its awful impact. This further look at the whole spectrum helps us to see that we are only one of the cogs in the wheel. The whole burden is not ours. Regular time out to hear about research and ways of working with sudden death are essential.

2. Life outside work

Sport, leisure, courses, and other ways of being distracted, are essential. Many critical care, high-tech units arrange theatre/concert visits, barbecues, and other social events. Yoga, massage and aromatherapy are considered as 'alternative' medicine and can work extremely well for some. We need to unwind in a way that is not at the expense of our families.

3. Ask for a move

A move from well-worn routines and to something less demanding may be necessary. This may involve a change of hours, and the change may be all the stimulus we need to see things differently. Working with a different type of client or with a longer or shorter transaction are options worth considering. The alternative to a move is working for a change in the situation we are in.

4. Encouraging support systems

One way of doing this may be by setting up groups within the area of work. The structure of the work may have to be changed to give space to allow this. Remind each other regularly to care and support one another — we need to do this because of the old problem of not recognising our own needs.

5. Difficulties and expected outcomes

Some patients, clients and relatives will not match up to our expectations of them. We are dealing with people, and must acknowledge their right to reject what we have an offer. Some people have resources within themselves or elsewhere to support them with their difficulties.

Sometimes, planned ways of working will have to be changed or disrupted. If we fail to recognise this, or become inflexible to the needs of people, we will feel let down and become disillusioned.

POST TRAUMATIC STRESS DISORDER

The article by Durham et al (1985) on the emotional response of medical personnel, police, firemen, paramedics and rescue workers emphasises the impact of disaster on personnel — 80% had at least one symptom of post traumatic stress disorder (PTSD). On-the-scene staff had significantly more symptoms than did hospital staff. This article was based on completed questionnaires returned after an apartment building explosion in Greenville, North Carolina.

There are some responses which are referred to as disaster syndrome or Post Traumatic Stress Disorder. This disorder can, of course, be any individual's response to a traumatic event.

Some of the more recent work on this problem has emerged as a result of effects on soldiers of the Vietnam war. Kolb (1986), for example, cites the long-term excessive mortality of those who served in the military during the Vietnam conflict. Suicide and road traffic accidents were the causes of death that increased in this section of the population. Kolb recommends that serious consideration be given to reports of the impaired psychosocial and health status of these men.

Whilst many of our clients have suffered a traumatic life experience, so have some emergency rescue personnel and people working in critical care. Once an unmanageable level for stress is reached, recognised patterns of response emerge:

Initial phase — impact and denial

Despite the media commonly showing an overt, noisy and dramatic response to trauma, the reality is usually the opposite. The response may be flat and full of denial, apparently lacking in awareness of the true nature of the event. The immediate focus is on survival. It could be argued that the denial is of benefit to the worker in that it prevents excessive fears overwhelming him.

Intermediate phase — confrontation and disorder

In this phase the worker recognises what has happened. We see him having left the denial behind and clearly confronting the disaster.

Sleep disturbances, nightmares and dreams become a disturbing part of this phase. Preoccupation with the event, flashbacks and intrusive thoughts are usually a feature. People become hypersensitive to sudden loud noises or bangs; you may notice this on an orthopaedic ward, where there are victims of road traffic accidents.

Being dependent on others makes the worker angry, and the anger is often directed towards colleagues or authority and the organisation. This anger can have a rebellious, adolescent nature about it. The opposite end of this scale is passive non-compliance.

Depression and guilt are often obvious components of this anger. The loss of relatives, friends or companions can produce guilt, and any elation at survival becomes the opposite — guilt at survival. A worker who becomes particularly helpful or co-operative, never complaining or showing dissent, may be making amends for having wrongfully survived.

Colleagues can help the worker at this stage by assisting him to begin the process of grieving and coping. The worker may need his colleagues' permission to express such feelings, especially the men, who may feel foolish about expressing sad emotions.

Final phase — readjustment and recovery

Here, the worker invests his energy towards the future, and leaves the role of the sick person behind. You notice an interest in others, and in the community at large. He begins to lose his dependency and takes control of his own life. After rumination over what he is now capable of doing, he becomes hopeful of making the adjustment.

In summary, then, the psychological sequelae to a traumatic event are divided into three phases:

1. Initial phase — impact and denial
2. Intermediate phase — confrontation and disorder
3. Final phase — readjustment and recovery.

Colleagues can help the carer by having insight into these phases and recognising where she is. They can then help her through the phases, to assist her in reaching her full potential again.

These are just a few suggestions for dealing with the symptoms of burnout and Post Traumatic Stress Disorder. We have looked at ways of working with and addressing difficulties within the individual.

We will now move on to setting up support systems within the organisation. The first one to consider is debriefing critical incidents.

STRESS DEBRIEFING

The recent spate of disasters has highlighted how the carer can become the victim. We have begun to recognise the phenomenon of bystander bereavement, i.e. not being a direct victim but witnessing a painful or traumatic event.

Working with sudden death may be just that; witnessing or being overwhelmed by the anguish of the people, at the time or later, and not having the resources or ability to prevent this somehow consuming us. The carer then becomes the victim.

In their study of one disaster, Durham et al (1985) indicated that 70% of the workers reported intrusive, repetitive thoughts about the event, and 15% reported intrusive dreams and depression. Workers who had been at the scene were more likely to experience these difficulties.

Adjustment in this study involved focusing on the meaning of the event, gaining mastery over the situation, and preparing mentally for a recurrence of the event. Each of these tasks is an issue for workers in any sudden death.

Many of the staff working with sudden death in these disaster areas report how surprised they are at their own calmness at the time. Woodruff (1989) reported that hours and days later, the stress became apparent. Vivid dreams, shaking, anxiety or not wanting to return home were some common responses. Although they were part of some major event, these were still sudden deaths in families, in individuals.

This study concluded that staff counsellors should be available for everyday hospital events that cause stress, not only of disasters.

What structured approaches are there to disastrous events? In my investigations over the past 2 years I have talked to people in the UK, Australia and the USA about structured ways of debriefing critical incidents (Wright 1989). Some of these incidents involved the death and injury of large numbers of people. Others, whilst not involving large numbers, concerned the sudden, maybe traumatic deaths of one or more people.

These deaths demanded from the health service and other personnel a sudden outpouring of resources both physically and emotionally. They are best described as critical incidents.

CRITICAL INCIDENTS

A critical incident is any situation, faced by emergency personnel, that causes them to experience unusually strong emotional reactions. These feelings have the potential to interfere with their ability to function at the time or later. Critical incidents result in some characteristic physical and psychological symptoms. This is quite normal and they are a common response to an abnormal event.

Some carers react immediately after the event or within a few hours or days. In some cases it is weeks or months before a reaction appears. The signs and symptoms of the stress reaction may last for a few days. Some support and understanding will often see the feelings dissipate.

For others, the event is so painful that more structured assistance is required. This is carried out most effectively by a peer group member with some skills in debriefing.

Critical Incident Stress Debriefing (CISD) is a skill in which the facilitator needs a good working knowledge of stress and counselling. Mitchell (1983) states that its value should not be underestimated as it prolongs the careers of personnel. This prevents resources having to be used on training new personnel and thus retains expertise. Mitchell describes this as a valuable commodity worth preserving.

Hearing too many expressions of pain, and witnessing too many broken bodies, may take its toll. The three frameworks used to alleviate the stress of critical incidents are defusing, demobilisation and debriefing.

Defusing

Defusing may best be described as a short type of crisis intervention for critical care staff and other emergency personnel. It is particularly suited to this group of people who are taught to act and control situations.

The aim of the defusing is to make the incident less harmful.

This is achieved by helping to restore control and by providing immediate support and assistance. It should reduce tension, focus on strengths and help carers to regain emotional control.

This focus on skills helps to ensure a return to normal functioning and the start of the process of recovery. A return to cognitive functioning enables the person to think rather than react.

The facilitator or interventionist maintains a low profile. The people involved should be encouraged to take the lead and do the talking. Once this process begins, most people become more spontaneous. Defusing is short term, and the parameters are set by the people themselves. They take charge of the level of emotional ventilation. They take it to where they want and then return to normal functioning.

Nurses will recognise how the report or handover time is used as a defusing period. Although the whole shift is to be reported on, or a group of patients in a certain order, any critical incident will receive the immediate attention. Until all the details of this event have been shared, it is difficult to discuss other events.

If attempts are made to prevent the incident being discussed until later, or in its exact chronological order, there will be difficulty in discussing other events. Attempts made to curtail the disclosure will cause it to emerge later. For any group of workers involved with a critical incident, time and attention are necessary to allow it to be laid to rest.

A satisfactory conclusion occurs when all the facts and feelings about the event have been shared. By putting it to rest in this way, a return to normal functioning is achieved. Key information is given to everyone so that the whole episode leaves no questions or perplexity. This allows a conclusion of the event.

The first 24 hours will see denial at its most powerful. This form of insulation may be necessary, and should not necessarily be viewed as unhealthy. It may be more appropriate to view denial in the long term as unhealthy.

A gentle approach to denial is always necessary, for in this impact phase denial may provide some safety, or a retreat from the pain and distress. This can be the safety valve needed for the moment. If it is persisting, this can be clarified later.

We must make a mental note of who may need more than defusing, and offer further help. A simple but powerful input at this time is to say 'Thank you'. Remind the workers that distress at such events is normal — it is the event and not they who are abnormal.

Some simple questions such as 'What happened there?' will elicit some facts about the incident, and 'What did you think about it?' encourages the sharing of thoughts. When you hear the answers, emphasise how normal they sound.

The aforementioned questions begin fairly safe disclosures. You can then begin to move more cautiously into what made the event different, and what was the worst part about it. What will help them most at this moment is something to help them manage their feelings. A question or statement that brings the span of duty to an end should close the defusing. This could be:

> 'Who will be at home when you get there?'

or

> 'It is now time to draw this to an end and for you to go home'.

This should take you naturally to the end of the defusing. Remember, it is a short act of discharge designed to help people return to cognitive functioning.

Demobilisation

Demobilisation provides personnel with a structured end to a span of duty. Large scale incidents benefit the most from this approach, so a room is needed for large numbers of personnel.

People entering the room should, ideally, be able to obtain a drink. As they will be tired, they will expect to be detained for 15 minutes at the most. The person leading the demobilisation should have as much accurate, factual information as is possible. There is no place for rumours or guesses.

Everyone should be ordered to attend the demobilisation, it is not just for the vulnerable or sensitive, or those who think they need it. It is for the whole team, and it should be made clear that they all need it. It is designed to facilitate an end to a stressful working period. The aims of demobilisation are:

1. To regain emotional control and cognitive functioning, and reduce tension.
2. To focus on strengths and skills, to re-evaluate the incident and receive some factual information.
3. To begin the recovery process and leave behind some of the stress.
4. To begin to be educated by the critical incident.

The process of demobilisation may be begun by the leader saying something like: 'At 15.30 today a multiple accident occurred on the southbound carriageway of the . . .'

All available information is then given as to rescue services and emergency personnel involved, numbers, types of casualties, and hospitals involved. Because different critical care staff may have looked after different members of a family, information about the condition of them all will be useful.

This helps to complete the picture for staff involved, and helps to prevent them taking away unanswered questions. The goals may seem similar to those of defusing; the difference is that demobilisation has a more definite time limit. The leader is clearly designated, and participation by staff is limited. They are told that further help may be given later, and where this may be obtained discreetly and with sensitivity.

The focus in demobilisation is primarily on cognitive functioning rather than emotional ventilation. The workers should be able to leave with a good knowledge of all available facts, and an overall perception of the event. Again, the expression of thanks and their dismissal help the personnel to bring the span of duty and the event to a conclusion.

At this stage you will want them to focus on their own resources. If the demobilisation is a positive experience, they will return for defusing or debriefing. The leader will still have to be available after the dismissal for people with immediate difficulties they cannot resolve themselves.

Large scale events involve many people, and you want to provide useful information in a short time to the maximum number of people. Assure them they did a good job, but that the event was abnormal and for this reason further help may be needed.

Critical incident stress debriefing (CISD)

This is the more formal type of debriefing, and should be done by someone with knowledge of counselling skills, stress management and, if possible, with a knowledge of the working procedure in an emergency situation. For example, if an emergency nurse is being debriefed, then an emergency nurse with the aforementioned skills would be ideal.

Formal CISDs take place 24–48 hours after the event. Mitchell (1983) says that a group meeting is most useful first, followed by individual, more formal debriefings.

The formal debriefing has six phases, which take a total of 3–5 hours:

Phase 1

After introductions, the rules about confidentiality are explained. The client needs an absolute assurance that no details of the debriefing will be divulged. If he feels guilty, particularly of some sin of omission rather than commission, he needs to be sure it will not be used against him.

Phase 2

The counsellor asks the client to give some details of personal involvement in the incident. He could describe what he saw, what he did, and what he heard and smelled. Anticipation of what will be encountered on arrival at the scene can be very distressing. Ask about how he received the message to attend, and about his thoughts prior to arriving on the scene.

Phase 3

When all this factual information has been dealt with you can go on to ask how he felt. This can centre around the questions:

'How did you feel at the time?'
'How are you feeling now?'
'Have you ever felt like this before?'

These questions usually produce a great outpouring of feelings; feelings of frustration, fear, guilt, anger and ambivalence are common. Many apologise that the feelings are about what appears to be a trivial aspect of the event. They need re-assurance about how it is important to them and therefore it needs to be expressed.

Phase 4

This phase concerns changes that have occurred both at the event and afterwards. Ask the client to tell you about the impact it has had on his life. Question him about what effect it will have on his future, and how it will alter it. The discussion should focus not only on the work situation, but on how it has affected him at home.

Phase 5

This phase is used to teach something about stress and how individuals respond. Information about common physical symptoms, sleep patterns and emotional reactions can be described. Again, the emphasis is on what happens to normal people, and that it was the event he was involved in that was abnormal and distressing.

Phase 6

This phase brings the debriefing to an end. It is aptly called the re-entry phase, because if debriefing has been effective, your client will be able to work again effectively. Hopefully, he will have discharged any distress, learned something about himself, and have been finally reassured.

When all outstanding issues are dealt with, the debriefing is clearly at an end. Any loose ends will have been tied up, and some people will talk of a plan of action which is now possible since they have been able to disengage from the critical incident.

CISD follow-up

After 6 months, the personnel may meet again as a group, but this is not always necessary. Some problem may have emerged, or re-emerged, because of the event. Individuals with long-term problems may also be identified here. Others will have been put in touch with some past conflict that compounded the difficulty. You may feel it needs further professional expertise or advice.

Many carers, social workers, crisis teams, as well as doctors and nurses, face people and incidents related to a disastrous event. Other incidents, whilst not a major disaster, are unusual or an exacerbation of a daily event.

A nurse, for example, may deal with a death from a road traffic accident daily, or quite frequently. Where there are two or three deaths in the same family or accident, the nurse will have to mobilise all her physical and emotional resources to deal with this. This can truly be described as a critical incident — it has the potential to leave the nurse feeling damaged and ineffective.

If people working with sudden death can be freed from guilt, anxiety and some frustration as well as other physical symptoms, that is good. It is good for their work, their efficiency and their effectiveness. Having to replace good personnel is a waste of resources and time.

With shortages of time, resources and personnel, we may have a long wait for debriefing to take place. Stress debriefing needs to be built into the structure and space of departments working with sudden deaths. It must be part of work schedules, and not an afterthought or something to be squeezed into too few hours in a day.

Some of the principles of debriefing are very simple. This simplicity may cause you to underestimate its value. If it is used well, there is every likelihood that some overwhelming and potentially destructive feelings will assume manageable proportions.

GROUP WORK AS A SUPPORT SYSTEM

Another support for people working with sudden death is to set time aside each week for the sole purpose of airing difficulties in a group. The fact that this can be done in working time has special implications. It is an acknowledgement by management that this work is stressful. It acknowledges the need to share, confront, comfort and support each other. This results in an effective and more cohesive team.

A multidisciplinary team recognises that everyone's contribution is valued and that common fears, anxieties and problems are shared. The group work endorses to other people and departments the value of the team's interaction, and is a good role model.

It will need to be made clear that there are benefits in sharing in this way. Many will wonder how safe it is to expose themselves to a group. It must be emphasised that the aim is to support each other, increase empathy and resolve emotional issues that occur due to the emotional nature of the work.

The sole aim of the group is to care for the staff. It is not to make them accountable, or increase their effectiveness, though the latter may be one of the spin-offs.

The group is simply a place to go and be yourself, with all your vulnerability. Hopefully, people will find solutions to

---

1. Everyone who is here belongs here just because he is here and for no other reason.
2. For each person, what is true is determined by what is in him, what he directly feels and finds making sense in himself and the way he lives inside himself.
3. Our first purpose is to make contact with each other. Everything else we want or need comes second.
4. We try to be as honest as possible and to express ourselves as we really are and really feel — just as much as we can.
5. We listen for the person inside, living and feeling.
6. We listen to everyone.
7. The group leader is responsible for two things only: he protects the belonging of every member, and he protects their being heard if this is getting lost.
8. Realism — if we know things are a certain way, we do not pretend they are not that way.
9. What we say here is confidential. No-one will repeat anything said here outside the group, unless it concerns only himself. This applies not just to obviously private things but to everything. If the individual concerned wants others to know something, he can always tell them himself.
10. Decisions made by the group need everyone taking part in some way.
11. New members become members because they walk in and remain. Whoever is here belongs.

Box 6.1 Ground rules for group sessions (Gendlin & Beebe 1968).

problems and will be able to air feelings and views in safety.

It may be necessary to define the aims of the group clearly and in a written form. Discussion could begin with people's expectations of the group. Another session may be spent discussing the ground rules of the group. I have found the ground rules of Gendlin & Beebe (1968) very useful. Anxiety will be reduced if everyone has a copy.

The overall philosophy of these rules emphasises how increased empathy can be achieved. They offer some clear guidelines about what is and what is not allowed.

Any organisational difficulties of the group, and a look at its aims and values, should be undertaken after 4–6 weeks.

The group facilitator will need specific skills, as well as a thorough knowledge of group processes and dynamics. Part of the group facilitator's role will be to offer information, though offering too much information, and with no thought for the timing, will cause people to drop out. Facilitating the group will be mostly concerned with sharing ideas, rather than with dispensing information.

Burnard (1987) suggests that verbal intervention, focussing on three different aspects of time, will be useful to the facilitator:

1. Clarifying recent talk
2. Developing current talk
3. Initiating further talk.

This framework is simply an easily retained way of managing the people in the group.

Group work should not be regarded as an economy of effort. It is an effective way of offering support and strength. It is not a way into individual counselling, or a substitute for this. Joining a group can give you the opportunity to give support as well as to receive it. This may cause the carers some problems. We find difficulty in receiving help, and even compliments.

On the other hand, we may take offered help although we do not need it, for fear of hurting the other person's feelings. We can be so defensive about being offered help that we reject it for reasons that are unfounded. We may, for example, find encouragement patronising, especially if people use inappropriate words or phrases like

'You have done that well.'
'What a good girl.'

Forming groups that only deal with a crisis denies the long-term difficulties of caring for people who are suddenly bereaved, and the toll it can take on staff. Space must therefore be made for these groups to meet in working time on a regular basis. The frequency will depend on the amount of work that involves sudden deaths.

Anxiety that sometimes people will have little to bring or say, or that they will be frantically searching for problems to make the group work, is usually unfounded. If the group facilitator makes it clear that good, positive, useful experiences can be brought to the group, this removes the idea that it is just for an outpouring of difficulties.

The group may simply want to sit and say quietly, away from the pressure of the work, how much they value each other, and their work, and why.

Staff counsellors

Some hospitals and organisations have made counsellors accessible to staff. More organisations have made counsellors accessible to staff more anonymously. Staff may contact the counsellor, who is independent of the organisation, and may visit the counsellor away from the place of work. For some people, this is the only safe way of receiving help, and this approach recognises that fact.

My only anxiety is that it puts the problems far away from the organisation, and it could be said that, by not having a resident staff counsellor in the vicinity of the work area itself, a major problem is hidden away. You will have to decide whether the positive outweighs the negative.

Supervision

Counsellors in any setting have long valued the concept and practice of supervision. Any carer who is very defensive about this must have her practice brought into question.

Supervision involves working with someone who is known for having skills, knowledge and experience in the practice of counselling. The supervisor is often senior in terms of years of experience in counselling. Supervision is distinguished from consultation by its ongoing process and the degree of intimacy with the supervisor.

One of the roles of the supervisor is to ensure that the counsellor or carer has the ability to work with the difficulties of the client. The nature of the relationship should provide an opportunity for personal and professional growth, but it is not in itself a therapeutic relationship.

Assisting the counsellor/carer to process usefully what she sees and hears, and how she responds to it, may be felt to be very confronting. There is no doubt that it is, and it may produce tension and some stress. This can and should be reduced to a working and productive level. It may involve the supervisor discussing the carer/counsellor's expectations about herself.

There are parallel experiential tasks in the supervisory and the therapeutic relationships. A working process, and the questions of what is productive, and how to establish rapport, are usefully explored in this way. The supervisor should be aware that there will be opportunities for role modelling. The carer/counsellor's receptiveness to feedback and its outcome is important.

The supervision may help to clarify immediate client problems and decision-making, which has a direct impact on the client. In an overview of a period of supervision, you may see its indirect impact on the client.

Although the accountability aspect of supervision is seen as a threat by some, it should be seen as a safeguard for both the client's and counsellor's interests. It often becomes apparent in these supervisory periods if the carer's stress is becoming intolerable.

Supervision is a way of caring for the carer.

The cost of caring can be too high. These are just a few responses to the stresses. It would seem, though, that we still cannot get it into our heads that prevention is better than cure.

REFERENCES

Bailey R D 1985 Coping with stress in caring. Blackwell Scientific, Oxford
Burnard P 1987 Developing skills as a group facilitator. The Professional
    Nurse 3: 1

Durham T W, McCammon S L, Allison E J 1985 The psychological impact of disaster on personnel. Annals of Emergency Medicine 14: 7
Gendlin E T, Beebe J 1968 An experimental approach to group therapy. Journal of Research and Development in Education 1: 19–29
Kolb L C 1986 Post traumatic stress disorder in Vietnam veterans. New England Journal of Medicine 314(10): 641–642
Manley K 1986 The dying patient in the intensive care unit — the problems. Care of the Critically Ill 2: 4
Melia K 1987 Everyday ethics for nurses. Nursing Times 83: 2
Mitchell J T 1983 When disaster strikes — the critical incident stress debriefing process. Journal of Emergency Services January
Pot-Mees C 1987 Beating the burnout. Nursing Times 83: 30
Woodruff I 1989 A report on staff reaction at Mayday University Hospital, following the major incident of the Purley train crash. British Journal of Accident and Emergency Medicine 4: 2
Wright B 1989 Critical incidents. Nursing Times 83: 19

Conclusion

My approach to working with sudden death is based on my 14 years' experience in an Accident and Emergency Department. This has involved me in the immediate crisis of sudden death and the care of relatives and friends of the deceased. It has also involved me in the care of ourselves as individuals and as a team.

Some of these families and individuals I have counselled in the long term, some ongoing from the point of death and others who have returned later, sometimes after a 6-month to 1-year period.

I enjoy this work and, as yet, have no wish to leave it. I believe that one of the reasons I have felt able to continue is because I have the opportunity to work with both ends of the spectrum of the loss. To have witnessed its painful beginnings, and followed people through the journey of making it manageable or otherwise, has taught me about the value of the carer.

It has also taught me about the adaptability and resourcefulness of each individual, and a great deal about familial and cultural responses.

Not many people have the opportunity of working in this way. It is rewarding and offers many opportunities for learning.

It is also stressful and painful, producing long periods of perplexity and a need to understand and philosophise. This aspect underlines the value of not being at work, and planning for and going on holiday.

I am constantly aware of the burden this work puts upon my wife, family and friends and, at times, myself. But mostly it is not like this, and I have met some unique and powerful people, some of whom I am happy to call my friends.

I feel I have to state my personal feelings and thoughts about working with sudden death because clients, friends and others often ask 'Why do you do it?' I am convinced that we can make a useful contribution at this most difficult time, though many will not need it and will not accept our offer of help.

There is plenty of work for us all to do. I know that when I and my contemporaries stop, others will be available to step in. I am not driven by a remorseless need to be in there amongst it all, and I hope I know when I have had enough, and will stop.

There are many structures available to help us in our interventions. I have described what I have found useful. It must be appreciated that my descriptions of how people responded at the time of the death and later, are my own interpretations of what I saw and heard.

The difficulties encountered in teaching and training for the work come from the experiences of myself and others. Having the opportunity to stand outside what I do, and examine its rewards and problems, is another reason why I can cope with it. In working with the stress of others as well as my own, I have been taught to cope with the work.

You will have gathered that, as well as having knowledge and skills learnt from teachers and experience, we need a personal philosophy if we are to work with sudden death and remain effective.

Here, I am re-evaluating mine. There is no end to it.

Bibliography

Bailey R D 1985 Coping with stress in caring. Blackwell Scientific, Oxford
Bowlby J 1981 Sadness and depression. Attachment and loss, vol 3.
    Penguin, Harmondsworth
Brewis T 1989 Stress and reactions of police officers when warning
    relatives of a sudden or unexpected death. Unpublished study for West
    Yorkshire Police for HND
Burnard P 1987 Developing skills as a group facilitator. The Professional
    Nurse 3: 1
Caplan G 1964 Principles of preventive psychiatry. Basic Books, New York
Cathcart F 1988 Seeing the body after death. British Medical Journal
    297: 997–998
Cook B, Phillips S G 1988 Loss and bereavement. Austin Cornish, London
DHSS What to do after a death
Doyle C J, Post H, Burney R E, Maino J, Keefe M, Rhee K J, 1987 Family
    participation during resuscitation: an option. Annals of Emergency
    Medicine 16: 6
Durham T W, McCammon S L, Allison E J 1985 The psychological impact of
    disaster on personnel. Annals of Emergency Medicine 14: 7
Durkheim E 1951 Suicide. The Free Press, New York
Freud S 1910 Two short accounts of psycho-analysis. Reprinted 1966.
    Penguin, Harmondsworth
Freud S 1917 Mourning and melancholia, standard edn, vol XIV. Hogarth,
    London
Gendlin E T, Beebe J 1968 An experimental approach to group therapy.
    Journal of Research and Development in Education 1: 19–29
Glick I O, Weiss R S, Parkes C M 1974 The first year of bereavement. John
    Wiley, New York
Henley S 1983 Bereavement by suicide. Bereavement care, vol 2. Cruse,
    London
Holmes T H, Rahe R H 1967 The social readjustment rating scale. Journal of
    Psychosomatic Research 11: 213

Jones W H, Buttery M 1981 Sudden death — survivors' perceptions of their emergency department experience. Journal of Emergency Nursing 7: 1

Kolb L C 1986 Post traumatic stress disorder in Vietnam veterans. New England Journal of Medicine 314(10): 641–642

Kübler-Ross E 1969 On death and dying. Macmillan, New York

Kübler-Ross E 1975 Death — the final stages of growth. Prentice Hall, New Jersey

Kübler-Ross 1978 To live until we say goodbye. Prentice Hall, New Jersey

Lindemann E 1944 Symptomatology and management of acute grief. American Journal of Psychiatry 101: 141–149

Lazarus R 1966 Psychological stress and the coping process. McGraw Hill, New York

Lundin T 1984 Morbidity following sudden and unexpected bereavement. British Journal of Psychiatry 144: 84–88

Manley K 1986 The dying patient in the intensive care unit — the problems. Care of the Critically Ill 2: 4

Melia K 1987 Everyday ethics for nurses. Nursing Times 83: 2

Mitchell J T 1983 When disaster strikes — the critical incident stress debriefing process. Journal of Emergency Services January

Onions C T 1983 The shorter Oxford English dictionary. Oxford University Press, Oxford

Otto H 1975 Holistic therapy. In: Harper R (ed) The new psychotherapies. Prentice Hall, New Jersey

Parkes C M 1975 Bereavement; studies of grief in adult life, 2nd edn. Penguin, Harmondsworth

Peppers L G, Knapp R J 1980 Motherhood and mourning. Praeger, New York

Pot-Mees C 1987 Beating the burnout. Nursing Times 83: 30

Raphael B 1980 Primary prevention — fact or fiction? Australian and New Zealand Journal of Psychiatry 14: 163–174

Raphael B 1984 The anatomy of bereavement — a handbook for the caring professions. Hutchinson, London

Raphael B 1986 When disaster strikes. Hutchinson, London

Shanfield S B, Benjamin G A H, Swain B J 1986 Parents' responses to the death of adult children from accidents and cancer: a comparison. American Journal of Psychiatry 141(9): 1092–4

Woodruff I 1989 A report on staff reaction at Mayday University Hospital, following the major incident of the Purley train crash. British Journal of Accident and Emergency Medicine 4: 2

Wordon J W 1983 Grief counselling and grief therapy. Tavistock, London

Wright B 1985 Hostility in accident and emergency departments. Nursing Mirror 161(4): 42–44

Wright B 1989 Critical incidents. Nursing Times 83: 19

Useful organisations for the bereaved

Compassionate Friends

5 Lower Clifton Hill
Clifton
Bristol BS8 1BT

0272 292738

Offers support and help for people suffering from the loss of a child. Leaflets available.

CRITECH — Crisis Counselling, Training, Education, Support, Information Service

Accident and Emergency
Leeds General Infirmary
Leeds LS1 3EX

0532 432799

Offers training, debriefing and an information service for those working with sudden death and other life crises.

Cruse — Bereavement Care

126 Sheen Road
Richmond
Surrey TW9 1UR

01-940–4818

3 Rutland Square
Edinburgh
Midlothian

031–229 6275

A counselling service with branches all over the UK. They have a wide range of literature.

Foundation for the Study of Infant Death

5th Floor
4 Grosvenor Place
London SW1 7HD

01–235 1721

Gay Switchboard

BM Switchboard
London WC1N 3XX

01–349 0839

Twenty-four hour help line for lesbians and gay men. Can refer to their bereavement project.

Jewish Bereavement Counselling Service

14 Chalgrove Gardens
London NW3 3PN

01–349 0839

Will send trained counsellors to bereaved people's homes. Operating only in Greater London but refers to other individuals in other areas.

The Lisa Sainsbury Foundation

8–10 Crown Hill
Croydon
Surrey

01–686 8808

Offers information and training support to those caring for the dying and the bereaved. Videos, literature and trainers can be made available to organisations.

St Christopher's Hospice Information Service

51–59 Lawrie Park Road
Sydenham
London SE26 6DZ

01–778 9252

Can provide information about approximately 90 hospices in the UK.

Stillbirth and Neonatal Death Society (SANDS)

Argyle House
29–31 Euston Road
London NW1 2SD

01–833 285

Advice and long-term support through local groups to newly bereaved parents of stillbirths and babies who die in the first month of life.

Support After Termination of Abnormality (SATFA)

22 Upper Woburn Place
London WC1H OEP

Support group run by women and couples who have experienced a termination of pregnancy because of abnormality.

Index